W0007826

"This amazingly well-organized, concise and informative book covers all aspects of having a baby from fertility issues to diet and nutrition, to the challenges and rewards of pregnancy, to life after baby comes. Though I've read countless books on the subject, have had a son and grandkids, and have helped numerous people have their own children, I was impressed by the wisdom, depth and detail of this book. It's warm, 'user friendly' and will certainly prove a great companion for the many people on the journey to parenthood."

- Rosemary Gladstar, herbalist and author of
Herbal Healing for Women *and* The Gladstar Family Herbal.

"Sarah, you are an angel! I have learned a lot of things that I need to change in my life. I do not feel helpless anymore. I thank God for people like you. One of these days, you will get an email from me, telling you that I am pregnant."

- a Mother-to-be

"Linda Page and Sarah Abernathy have produced an important and thorough book on attaining a healthy pregnancy with a natural approach to many pregnancy problems. A must for families to be."

- Elson M. Haas, MD (www.elsonhaas.com), Integrated Medicine Practitioner, author of Staying Healthy with Nutrition *and many other books.*

"As a doula and mother of two, I'm always looking for responsible information on pregnancy, childbirth and breastfeeding challenges. *Do You Want to Have a Baby?* presents quality natural health advice that parents can use with confidence. I would recommend this book to my clients."

- Michele Nizza, B.A., C.M.T., C.L.C., C.D. (Doulas of North America)

"Linda, I'm a brand new student at Clayton College working on my BS in Holistic Nutrition. I'm really enjoying your *Healthy Healing* book, which is one of my study guides for Introduction to Natural Health. I share it daily with my daughter, mother and sister and encourage them to use the natural approach to healing. Thanks again."

- Robin H.

Books by Dr. Linda Page

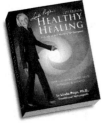

Healthy Healing, 12th Edition
The Ultimate Resource For Improving Your Health Naturally

In its first edition nearly 20 years ago, Dr. Linda Page's book, Healthy Healing, was the only one of its kind. Now updated and expanded, Healthy Healing is still the easiest to use bestselling natural health reference book on the market.

Customize your own personal healing program using natural therapies for more than 300 ailments through diet, whole herb supplements and exercise.

12th Edition, 664 Pages, Illustrated, 1884334-92-X SRP: $32.95
Spiral Bound Edition - 1884334-93-8 SRP: $35.95

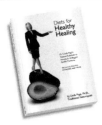

Diets for Healthy Healing
Natural Solutions to America's 10 Biggest Health Problems

Food is powerful medicine. Sometimes it's your best medicine… even for difficult diseases. Linda Page, America's foremost nutrition and herb expert, has worked with this healing principle for over two decades and has written this book as your primary guide to using food as your best medicine. In Diets for Healthy Healing, each chapter reviews a health problem and provides an easy-to-follow nutrition plan. Healing recipes, nutritional supplements, whole herbs, bodywork and exercise recommendations are included as part of the healing program.

1st Edition, 256 Pages, Illustrated, 1884334-83-0 SRP: $18.95

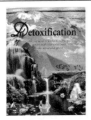

Detoxification
Recharge and Rejuvenate Your Body, Mind and Spirit!

More than 25 thousand new toxins enter our environment each year. Detoxification is a necessary commitment for staying healthy in a destructive world. In this complete guide of detailed instructions for detoxification and cleansing, Dr. Page shows you: what you can expect when you detox; what a good cleanse really does; how to direct a cleanse for best results; and much more!

264 Pages, Illustrated, 1884334-54-7 SRP: $21.95

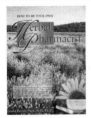

How To Be Your Own Herbal Pharmacist
108 Step-by-Step Healing Formulas!

Formulating herbal combinations is usually a deep dark secret between herbalists. Most books on herbs don't really show you how to combine herbs to address specific ailments. This fascinating book shows you how it's done, with detailed work pages, how to take the formula for best results, and much more!

2nd Edition, 256 Pages, Illustrated, 1884334-78-4 SRP: $18.95

This book is dedicated to all of the hopeful parents around the world, who know that to create and nurture a new life is one of the most treasured gifts Nature offers us.

This book is also dedicated to the wonderful world of babies. At first glance, babies are so dependent on us. But let us never underestimate their resiliency and how, in the end, we are much more dependent on them than they are on us.

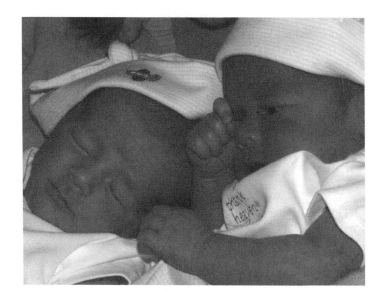

Acknowledgments

This book has been a wonderful conception and birthing project of its own. I'd like to thank everyone involved for making it possible, including:

Linda Page for all of the creative insight and natural health wisdom she has graciously shared with me over the years. Thank you for introducing me into this field of helping others and helping myself.

Elliot Page for all of his practicality and attention to key details, like book distribution and "keeping the lights on." I don't thank you enough for everything you do.

Leah Thomson-Vizcaino for her marketing expertise and her thoughtful sharing of her own very special pregnancy experience. Your strength of character during these last 9 months has taught me so much. Thanks for being such a willing pregnancy product sampler!

Michael Kohler for his calm presence and dedication in the undertaking of the layout and design for this book. Without you, this beautiful baby book wouldn't be born! Special thanks to Amber Kohler for her thoughtful input and sense of humor during our Healthy Healing working lunches and brainstorming meetings.

Darlene Matsumoto for her dedicated research, attention to detail and heartfelt desire to get the best information out to the people who really need it.

The entire HEALTHY HEALING staff, Jim, Robert, Crystal, Victor and Omar for their support over these last months as I've buried myself in the writing of this book. Special thanks to all of our sales representatives for continuing to share our Healthy Healing message around the country.

Our new partners, Brent Johnson, Luke Petterson, Bernard Hicks and Todd Bassinger, for their steadfast belief in our company, this book and all of the families who have requested it.

Our professional colleagues who generously donated pregnancy, breastfeeding and baby care samples for Leah to try during this book's gestation period: All One Nutrition, American Health/Home Health, Barleans Organic Oils, Jason Naturals, Earth Mama Angel Baby, Health from the Sun, Maitake Products, Motherlove, Mother's Intuition, Noveya, Pure Essence Labs, Wellements and more.

Talented midwives and doulas everywhere for sharing their vast pregnancy/childbirthing expertise with so many women. Their hard won experiences have paved the way for women everywhere to take back control over their bodies.

My wonderful family: my parents Mary Abernathy, Walter Abernathy, my stepmother, Nancy Abernathy, my sisters Emily and Beth, and my brother Gregg. My wonderful second family: Marilyn and John Anton, and my fiance, Nick. I love you all.

All of my fantastic friends, you know who you are. I thank God for you every day.

And finally, to you reading this book, it is my great hope that you will reap the fertility benefits of a healthy lifestyle and that your dreams for a family will be fulfilled.

Love,

Sarah Abernathy

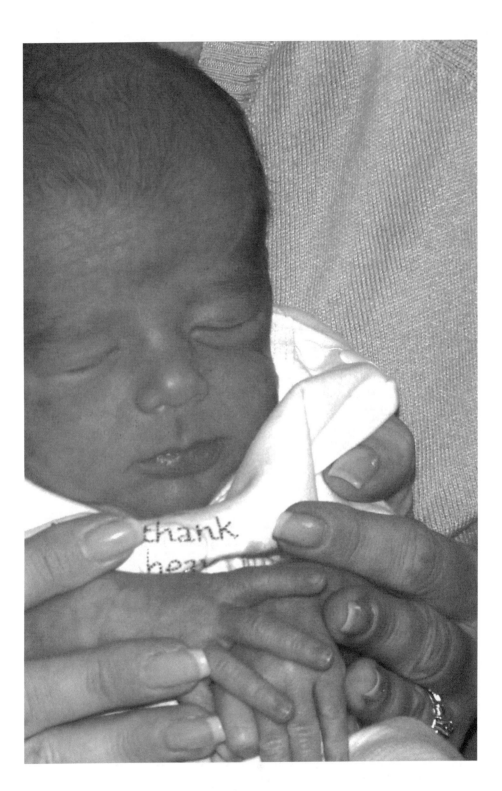

do you want to have a Baby?

Natural Fertility Solutions and Pregnancy Care

by Sarah Abernathy, Herbal Consultant
and Linda Page, Ph.D., Traditional Naturopath

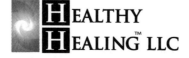

HEALTHY HEALING™ LLC

This reference is to be used for educational information. It is not a claim for cure or mitigation of disease, but rather an adjunctive approach, supplying individual nutritional needs that otherwise might be lacking in today's lifestyle.

First Edition, September 2006

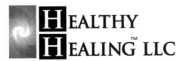

HEALTHY
HEALING™ LLC

Copyright © September 2006 by Sarah Abernathy and Linda Page.
Published by Healthy Healing Enterprises LLC
www.healthyhealing.com

Cover and book design by Michael Kohler.

Publisher's Cataloging-in-Publication
(Provided by Quality Books, Inc.)

Abernathy, Sarah.
    Do you want to have a baby? : natural fertility
solutions and pregnancy care / by Sarah Abernathy and
Linda Page.
    p. cm.
    Includes bibliographical references and index.
    ISBN 1-884334-39-3

    1. Pregnancy. 2. Infertility. 3. Naturopathy.
4. Herbs--Therapeutic use.   I. Rector-Page, Linda G.
II. Title.

RG525.A23 2006   618.2
                           QBI06-600145

Contents

Chapter 2

Enhancing fertility, naturally - 32

Chapter 3

Overcoming sexually transmitted diseases & reproductive blockages - 48

Chapter 4

Miscarriage prevention – how to improve your chances - 66

Chapter 5

Pregnancy after 40 - the challenges and the rewards - 74

Chapter 6

Pregnancy and prenatal tests - 77

Chapter 7

Optimal eating for two (or more) - 82

Chapter 8

Natural pre-natal care: targeted herbs and supplements for a mother-to-be - 92

Chapter 9
Premature labor and birth - 96

Chapter 10
Herbs for a healthy pregnancy - 100

Chapter 11
Special problems during pregnancy - 111

Chapter 12
Bodywork for two - 127

Chapter 13
It's getting to be time - 132

Chapter 14

About breast feeding - 143

Chapter 15

After your baby is born - 150

Afterword by Leah Thomson-Vizcaino:

Foreword By Leah Thomson-Vizcaino

Reflections on the journey to Motherhood

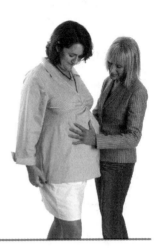

So you want to have a baby? How about two? You never know what you are going to get. Well, we wanted to have a baby, but were a little naive about the whole process.

I had never been pregnant before, so I made a lot of incorrect assumptions from the beginning, starting with telling my husband not to worry about going to the doctor with me on that first visit. (This was one of the dumber things I have done.) I figured they were just going to make me pee in a cup and tell me that I was pregnant. Little did I know that they would hook me right up to the ultrasound machine and show me not one baby, but two little people growing inside of me. My husband really should have been there to experience the shock and excitement of that precious moment. Instead I handed him the ultrasound photo with no explanation and, shocked, he exclaimed, "Oh my God, there's two!"

Being pregnant with twins has been a wonderful, exciting, and scary experience filled with so many emotions. One minute you are happy and excited, and the next minute you are scared to death and wondering how you are going to care for, much less pay for these little people. That being said, I don't recommend going to see your accountant before you conceive. I can't imagine that it would help your fertility, and it is probably unnecessarily frightening.

I think almost every single assumption I made about pregnancy was either wrong, or completely off base.

For example:

I assumed… it would take us much longer to get pregnant. I am 35 and my husband is 37. To the best of my knowledge, neither he nor I had ever been pregnant or impregnated anyone, so this was new territory for us.

In reality… It took unprotected baby making love for approximately 2 months before we conceived. Wow, that CRYSTAL STAR CONCEPTIONS™ TEA really worked.

I assumed… I would be one of the many women whose pregnancy ends in miscarriage. My Mom had put a little of the fear of God in me about waiting to tell people about my pregnancy until after the first trimester. She had a miscarriage, and then a baby, then another miscarriage and then another baby, so I figured my fate would be similar.

In reality… I am currently 5 months pregnant with twins, and so far so good. I am having a very healthy pregnancy.

I assumed… I would have no problem brushing my teeth. The kids are growing in my uterus not my mouth.

In reality… The entire first trimester, the minute I stuck my toothbrush in my mouth my gag reflex was activated. It lasted for about two months. One time, brushing my teeth triggered a gag reflex and made me vomit. It happened so quickly that I had to throw up in the sink because I couldn't make it to the toilet. That's what I call lightening fast vomit!

I assumed… with twins I would experience more extreme pregnancy symptoms.

In reality… my pregnancy symptoms have been pretty minor so far. I had very little morning sickness, two weeks of sensitivity to smell, but my heartburn has been pretty bad. No cravings to speak of except for milk. I really craved milk.

I assumed… I would get hemorrhoids after I had the babies, not during pregnancy.

In reality… Okay, when you're pregnant you sometimes get constipated. Well, lucky me, I got a nice dose of hard to heal hemorrhoids. They're not painful, but definitely irritating.

I assumed… I would get that "pregnancy glow" that people talk about.

In reality… The glow in my case seems to be due to an excessive amount of oil production, and all I seem to be getting is hormonal acne on my neck and around my lips. (This is not my idea of attractive.)

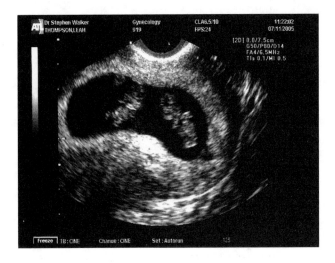

I seem to get asked the same questions over and over again. Are you going to breastfeed? Are you going to deliver the babies vaginally? My standard answer is, "I am going to try."

I, like most pregnant women would like very much to deliver my babies vaginally, but since twin births are considered high risk, they have you deliver in a surgical room just in case there are any problems. My doctor says that I have a 70% chance of delivering vaginally.

Regarding breastfeeding, I am going to do everything in my power to breastfeed, but honestly I am nervous about breastfeeding two babies. I worry that I won't have enough milk to go around. I already have a wonderful supplement company who has offered to provide me samples of an herbal tea to enhance my milk production.

The pregnancy experience is making my husband and I process a ton of different emotions, but ultimately it's bringing us much closer together. Watching your body change is a very surreal experience. My breasts seem like they are enormous and my stomach doesn't feel that far behind my breasts. I find myself looking at my growing belly in the mirror and thinking, "little people are growing in there." It's such an amazing thing!

So, you still want to have a baby? Congratulations and read on. You're sure to find information that will be helpful throughout your fertility and pregnancy journey. Some of the tips in this book come directly from my own pregnancy experience here at HEALTHY HEALING, including my favorite pregnancy supplements and the health advice that has worked the best for me.

Introduction

Having a baby is one of Nature's greatest miracles. Pregnancy, childbirth and parenting are experiences of a lifetime. For many women and their partners, pregnancy is a time of enhanced creativity, new perspective and awe at the wonder of life. I believe that parenthood is a divinely inspired gift. You must cherish and use it wisely if you have been blessed enough to receive it.

You may be reading this book because you've discovered getting pregnant or staying pregnant is difficult. Today conception eludes many otherwise healthy adults. Our modern lifestyle adds to the problem with its surplus of chemicals that affect male and female fertility, and even the fertility of future generations. In addition, there is no question that more and more women are opting for later life pregnancies to establish their careers before starting their families. While from a medical perspective it is the best time ever in history to have a child later in life, pregnancy after 40 creates new challenges.

Pregnancy at any age presents physical and mental challenges. The female body must change tremendously to meet the needs of a developing child. Weight gain, food cravings, morning sickness, complexion changes, fatigue, even vision problems can occur during pregnancy. Further, natural childbirth is called labor for a good reason; it's hard work. Yet, the female body is designed with exactly this purpose in mind.

This book is intended to guide you through the journey of healthy conception and pregnancy, naturally. It serves as a guide to healthy eating and living for women and men who are struggling with fertility problems or who are already using conventional fertility treatments. It explores the entire gambit of pregnancy and childbirth challenges, including information on reducing miscarriage risk, presenting safe, natural options that can help get you through the experience of pregnancy more comfortably with a healthy, happy baby.

Natural therapies are ideally suited for special problems during pregnancy and for infertility problems. The majority of infertility problems can be solved through lifestyle changes, use of supportive herbs and supplements, and increased education about you and your partner's fertility status. Sometimes all that is needed to overcome an infertility problem is a more relaxed attitude, a renewed partnership with your spouse, and a little time. Further, a balanced, nutritious diet is important for fertility and during pregnancy, a time when nutrient demands are higher than ever. Making the decision to start a family with your partner is a major commitment and one I believe you should make with your best health in mind.

In addition, expectant dads need to prepare for many changes. Instead of feeling left out or ignored, embrace your newfound parenthood by participating in childbirth education or Lamaze classes with your spouse. While this book does not address the unique issues that affect couples in same-sex relationships who hope to have or adopt children, I hope these men and women will benefit from this book as a guide to a healthy lifestyle and diet for all hopeful parents-to-be.

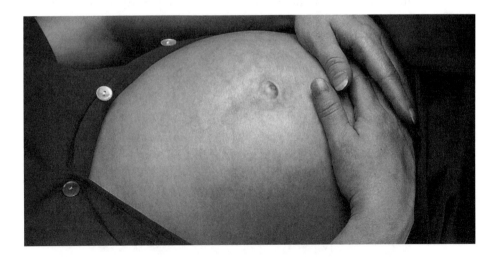

Chapter One

What's your fertility status?

In America, 20% of married couples of child-bearing age have trouble conceiving and completing a successful pregnancy. The latest statistics show that around one in five U.S. couples is "infertile," which means that they have tried unsuccessfully to become pregnant for at least one year. The fertility industry is big business, grossing $2 billion a year. Fertility problems are complex and usually correctable without invasive procedures or fertility drugs. Nutritional, environmental, biological and social factors are all involved in fertility problems. And there are different stages and levels of fertility that can be enhanced through simple, natural means.

Nutritionally, our diets are still lackluster, with an abundance of fats, sugars and processed foods forming the basis for the meals many of us eat on a daily basis. Nature tries to avoid conception under conditions of inadequate nutrition or obesity. Environmentally, we're exposed to more toxic chemicals than any other generation, and many of these chemicals are known hormone disrupters that can affect ovulation and lower sperm count!

Biologically, more women are struggling with reproductive blockages like fibroids, adhesions and endometriosis that can impede conception efforts. Further, years of oral contraceptive use has led to disruption of normal ovulatory cycles for many women. In these cases, the body may need up to a 1 year off the Pill to come back into a healthy balance. And, both men and women are facing an epidemic of Sexually Transmitted Diseases, some of which can lead to sterility and increased risks during childbirth.

Socially, men and women are waiting longer than ever to start their families and family roles are changing dramatically. More women are becoming primary breadwinners for their families. As a result, working women are waiting to have children until in their mid 30's and 40's, when fertility is no longer at its peak. Further, the U.S. is notoriously behind the times compared to the rest of the world when it comes to allowing working moms an appropriate amount of time off before returning to work to care for their newborns. Family planning has become more challenging than ever.

In spite of these factors, there is plenty of good news. You shouldn't panic if you don't conceive right away. There's only a 20-25% chance of successful conception during any monthly cycle. Just 60% of couples conceive within the first 6 months of trying. 90% conceive within 18 months. More good news: Recent research suggests that while pregnancy risks do increase with age, they remain quite small. 1 in 5 women having a first child in the U.S. is over 35.

Many so called "infertile" couples have gone on to become parents by making healthy lifestyle changes and using natural therapies. Up to 45% of couples conceive after discontinuing their fertility treatments! So, try not to get discouraged if you don't conceive right away.

The world of fertility technology

Fertility research and treatment has grown leaps and bounds over the last thirty years. Today's treatments offer hope for people who thought they would never be able to conceive. New fertility technologies have clearly opened new doors to couples who want options for later life pregnancies. Still, treatments are prohibitively expensive for most of us, and are only beginning to be eligible for insurance coverage. In addition, as with all drugs and medical procedures, fertility treatments can cause side effects and body trauma.

While this book focuses on natural therapies for enhanced fertility and healthy pregnancy, here is a short overview of some of the medical fertility treatments in use today and what you can expect from them:

• **In vitro fertilization,** first used in 1978, is the most common infertility treatment in use today. More than 250,000 babies have been born as a result of IVF. Success rates are continuing to improve. In IVF, the egg and sperm are introduced for possible fertilization in a lab. Eggs that are successfully fertilized are transferred into a woman's uterus, with a 10-40% chance of progressing into a normal pregnancy. Fertility drugs are used with IVF to stimulate the ovaries to produce several eggs for fertilization. There are precautions with IVF treatments. A 1999 study in the journal Lancet shows women treated with fertility drugs have twice the risk of developing breast cancer - and over 5 times the risk for uterine cancer as other women. Another study shows women who have not been pregnant before increase their risk for ovarian cancer 27 times when they use fertility drugs. Moreover, women report drug side effects like mood swings and chronic bloating. Many couples use donor sperm or eggs to avoid these side effects. Still, even in these cases, IVF treatments can cause multiple pregnancies with possible complications. A new technique called "blastocyst transfer" is sometimes used today with IVF to reduce risk of multiple pregnancies and improve the chances of having a successful pregnancy. Blastocyst transfer implants use embryos that have developed for five days after fertilization. Embryos at this stage are stronger, and have a higher probability of proceeding into a healthy fetus.

Good news: starting April 2005, the NATIONAL HEALTH SERVICE has started funding one IVF cycle for couples experiencing fertility problems, depending on your age and where you live. The news comes as a big relief for many hopeful parents. IVF costs up to $15,000 per procedure!

• **Gamete intrafallopian transfer (GIFT),** combines eggs from a woman's ovaries with a man's sperm in a flexible tube that is then injected into the fallopian tubes, allowing fertilization to take place more naturally in the woman's body. However, this type of fertility treatment requires a woman to undergo two separate procedures, putting her body under more stress, and, like IVF, GIFT can result in multiple pregnancies. One drawback: if a viable pregnancy doesn't occur with a GIFT treatment, it's not possible to tell if the egg and sperm were compatible or if fertilization occurred at all.

• **Zygote intrafallopian transfer (ZIFT),** combines the principles of IVF and GIFT. Eggs and sperm are mixed outside of the body. The fertilized eggs are then returned to the fallopian tubes, through which they travel to the uterus.

• **Intracytoplasmic Sperm Injection (ICSI),** introduced in 1993 to help improve fertility for subfertile men, involves the injection of a single sperm directly into an egg for placement into the fallopian tubes or the uterus. It's used in conjunction with IVF. Some research shows ICSI may cause abnormalities in embryos and even slow development in children.

How to determine your most fertile periods

If you're a woman reading this book, chances are that you already know that you're most fertile during ovulation. Ovulation refers to the period of time during the menstrual cycle when the ovaries release a mature ovum (egg) for fertilization. You can significantly increase your chances of becoming pregnant by having sex right before and after ovulation. There are many effective methods to predict ovulation. First, look for ovulation body signs. Many women experience light cramping during ovulation, called intermenstrual pain. There are also clear changes in cervical fluid to watch for (see next page). The following methods can empower you in your conception efforts.

Tip for getting pregnant? After having sex, stay in bed with your legs elevated on a pillow with the man's semen inside you for about 20 minutes. Most women instinctively head to the bathroom after sex to clean up. But, this can be counterproductive to sperms' valiant effort to reach your egg!

Ovulation tests: Available over-the-counter, ovulation tests predict your fertility through urine testing at specific times of day. They work by detecting the surge of luteinizing hormone (LH) that occurs just prior to ovulation (approximately 24-36 hours) in your urine. Your most fertile period is on the day your LH surge is detected, and the day after. Ovulation tests are usually reliable and inexpensive, and offer couples a day or more to plan for intercourse.

Ovulation calculator: In a normal menstrual cycle, ovulation most commonly occurs between day 5 and day 15. One easy way to try to calculate when you're ovulating is by subtracting 14 to 16 days from the date of your next period. There are many good ovulation calculators online today. Check out *www.webmd.com* and *www.4women.gov*. Note: Some women's fertile periods are unpredictable. If your menstrual cycle is irregular, less than 21 days, or more than 35 days, an ovulation calculator will not be a good predictor of your most fertile periods. Work with a physician or use ovulation tests if this is the case for you to help determine your fertile periods.

Basal Body Temperature (BBT): BBT refers to your body temperature first thing when you wake up in the morning. Before ovulation, your temperature ranges from 97.2° to 97.7° before ovulation. In the two to three days before ovulation, expect a temperature rise of .5 to 1.6 degrees, a sign of ovulatory hormonal changes. When your temperature goes up, it's a good time to try to conceive. For the most accurate results, take your BBT before you get out of bed or brush your teeth with a special BBT thermometer available at pharmacies. For more information on BBT testing, visit *www.early-pregnancy-tests.com*.

Cervical mucous changes: We tend to think of vaginal discharge as a sign of yeast or bacterial infection, and it certainly can be. However, some types of vaginal discharge are perfectly normal, and an indicator of your most fertile periods. You can check your own cervical mucous by swabbing the area with a little toilet tissue or clean finger. During non-fertile times, cervical mucous is usually light or sticky. During fertile times, cervical mucous is usually clear and slippery, like the texture of an egg white. Experts say you are most fertile the last day you experience this type of cervical mucous.

Home saliva tests: Home saliva tests are another option to help you determine your most fertile periods. These types of tests require that you examine monthly changes in your saliva patterns (you can also use cervical mucous) under a special microscope. I've tried this method, but found the patterns to be difficult to decipher with any certainty of accuracy. I prefer the previous four methods. Still, viewing the slides can be a useful tool for many women.

When ovulation is unpredictable

During puberty, young women have up to 300,000 eggs in their ovaries. With this seemingly endless supply of eggs, it's surprising that there is any decline in female reproductive capacity at all. But for each egg that matures and is released during the menstrual cycle, another 500 eggs are absorbed by the body. Beginning as early as the mid 30's, egg quality begins to decline and many women no longer ovulate every month. As egg supply lessens or is of poorer quality, Nature offers fewer opportunities for conception.

By the time a woman reaches menopause, she usually has only several thousand remaining eggs, most of which are no longer suitable for fertilization. Preliminary animal research suggests it may be possible to produce more eggs than one is born with. Perhaps as technology and reproductive knowledge advances, the concept of "old eggs" as a cause of infertility will no longer be relevant. For now, it is far too early in the research to know how much it could benefit older women who still want to have children. Nature never does anything by whimsy; pregnancy and childbirth during menopause may never have been part of her reproductive plan for us.

Problems with ovulation can occur long before menopause. Harvard research shows that up to 31% of premenopausal women fail to ovulate at any point during their menstrual cycles. Environmental factors may be involved in this drop in fertility and the problem may start as early as in the womb. Evidence suggests exposure to hormone mimicking pesticides and chemicals (xenoestrogens) in the womb damages ovarian follicles. Respected hormone expert, John Lee M.D. believed it could even result in an inability to ovulate or produce enough progesterone for conception later in life (luteal phase failure).

Too much or too little body fat also affects hormone production and can hinder ovulation. In one study published in the journal *Fertility and Sterility*, weighing 85% or less of ideal weight was linked to a five-fold increase in infertility due to ovulation problems. Weighing 120% or more of ideal weight doubled infertility risk.

Smoking also damages and ages a woman's reproductive system. A major Dutch study reveals that smoking adds the equivalent of 10 years to a woman's reproductive age and can significantly reduce chances of success in IVF treatments.

A midwife's advice... before modern times, ovulation was triggered by the monthly pattern of dark nights interrupted by three nights of light from the full moon. Modern conveniences like electricity mean most women today sleep in rooms with some lights from clocks or night lights, which may disrupt normal ovulation patterns. You can help stimulate ovulation every month by keeping your room very dark for the first two weeks and then sleeping with a night-light on for three nights.

Is there a peak fertility time for men? Early research says yes! A recent Italian study shows a man's sperm count increases from 20 million to 25 million in the early evening, increasing chances of conception by 25%.

Seasonal fertility trends

Nature plays a powerful role in the timing of conception. Seasonal trends from around the world show that the best months for conception are early winter to early spring with November being the "peak" fertility month for both sexes. Research shows men's semen quality and quantity varies throughout the year and is at its highest potential for conception during these months. It is theorized that during winter, the pineal gland may be more active and a woman's endometrium (uterine lining) becomes more receptive for a fertilized egg. Nature, in her wisdom, may be encouraging our fertility at these times, as part of her divine plan for us and our planet's future.

Infertility factors

A common denominator for infertility for both sexes is too much free radical activity in the body from chemical exposure, hormone disruption, and poor nutrition. Infertility problems are about equally divided between men (about 35–40%) and women (over 35–40%). In 20–30% of cases, both the man and woman have fertility problems. In other cases, infertility has no known medical cause. Here's what we know about what's causing infertility challenges today:

Male Infertility, Subfertility and Poor Sperm Motility

Today twenty million U.S. men are characterized as semen infertile. Millions more are described as semen sub-fertile. Poor sperm motility (rather than low sperm count) affects about 10% of infertile men. Further, while age does not impact male fertility to the extent that it does female, a gradual lessening of semen quality does occur for men each decade after age 40. Testosterone levels also start to decline around age 40, falling up to 10% each decade. This phenomenon, called "andropause" is now recognized by almost eight in ten family physicians as a real condition that affects quality of life for men. Still, while today's men face clear fertility challenges, evidence suggests that the medical guidelines used to classify men's fertility are actually inaccurate.

Apart from the more common problems of low sperm count and motility, men's infertility can also be caused by sickle cell anemia, metabolic disorders, testicular cancer or trauma, undescended testes, anatomical obstructions, and varicocele (abnormally dilated testicular veins which affect sperm production). 19 to 41% of infertile men have a varicocele which may require medical treatment for reversal. Some herbs can decrease varicocele. See pg. 46-47 for more information. Chronic sexually transmitted infections can lead to scarring that affects men's fertility, too. See pg. 48 for more on STDs and fertility.

The Chemical Link to Male Infertility

A healthy human male produces about 1500 sperm with every heartbeat. However, worldwide studies show sperm counts have dropped on average by more than half over the last 50 years (one report from Britain shows a drop of 160 per milliliter to 66 million per milliliter). Sperm are rich in lipids, highly sensitive to free radical damage from toxic chemicals and pollutants. In one study, high free radical levels in the male reproductive tract was linked to infertility in 40% of men. In another study, a significant decline of sperm quality was seen in men with high exposure to three pesticides: alachlor, diazinon and atrazine, all commonly found in today's water supplies.

Long term exposure to solvents like paint, printing presses, and dry cleaning chemicals is also linked to male infertility. Over 1,000 workplace chemicals have been linked to reproductive problems. Exogenous estrogens from pesticides can lower sperm count, affect sperm viability and reduce the amount of seminal fluid produced by men. The highest risk jobs studied were: livestock and dairy farmers, fruit and flower growers, and gardeners. Men who work in plastic production, welding or who work with lead or other heavy metals face reproductive hazards, too.

Zinc is Critical to Male Fertility

The mineral zinc is crucial for male reproductive health. Zinc is involved in sperm formation and motility, and testosterone metabolism, too. Low zinc levels reduce both testosterone levels and seminal volume. Low prostate zinc levels have especially been connected to prostate cancer. My first suggestion to men dealing with fertility problems or sexual dysfunction is to eat more zinc-rich foods like fish and seafood (especially shellfish like oysters), seeds (sunflower, pumpkin and caraway), nutritional yeast, eggs, mushroom and wheat germ. Zinc can even enhance fertility for men who smoke by helping to offset the overload of heavy metals like cadmium in cigarettes. Zinc supplementation also improves sperm motility. For dosage and suggestions, see pg. 34.

What other nutritional and lifestyle factors reduce male fertility?

A fast-food diet high in trans fat and low in protective antioxidants decreases male fertility. Deficiencies of vitamin C and E are linked to male fertility problems. Too much workplace stress is a fertility blocker for men. Research from the University of Calgary shows men with the most daily work stress produce 1/3 less sperm than men under low stress. Heavy drinking and recreational drug use are other factors in low sperm count, sperm abnormalities and decreased sexual performance. Smoking is a major infertility factor that reduces the ability of sperm to bind to an egg. As with women, being overweight or underweight can also lead to fertility problems in men.

Boxers or Briefs? The scientific jury is still in disagreement on this one. Still, most reproduction experts will tell you that wearing loose fitting underwear is the best choice for a man's fertility. Researchers theorize too tight fitting underwear (like briefs) may raise body temperature and reduce viable sperm. It's probably smart to avoid prolonged exposure to heat from hot tubs and long bike rides while you're trying to have a baby.

Female Infertility: The Role of Aging and Reproductive Blockages

For women, hormone imbalance, an aging egg supply and reproductive blockages are the biggest conception inhibitors. Women's infertility is commonly caused by a problem with ovarian function (luteal phase failure), believed by some experts to be a result of exposure to estrogen-mimicking chemicals in the womb and progesterone deficiency. Hormone imbalance problems like polycystic ovary syndrome (PCOS) and fibroids routinely lead to fertility problems women. Low estrogen, associated with low body weight, is a known conception inhibitor.

A blockage in the fallopian tubes can also lead to female infertility. Fallopian tube blockage is usually caused by scar tissue from chronic pelvic infections or endometriosis, or accumulated fluid (hydrosalpinx). Minor fallopian tube blockages can usually be corrected through surgery. Massage therapy, acupuncture and physical therapy can decrease fallopian adhesions and improve reproductive function. See pg 38-41 for more.

Could you have a sperm allergy? Some women suffer from an immune response to their partners' sperm which prevents pregnancy. Unfortunately, there are no real symptoms for this condition except unexplained infertility. Some women say a sperm allergy causes a burning sensation, frequent UTI's or yeast infections after intercourse. Still, in these cases, there are often other medical causes. Some cases of sperm allergy cannot be explained, but in other cases a man's previous vasectomy and vasectomy reversal may play a role. Almost all men who undergo a vasectomy (surgical operation that causes sterility) will produce antisperm antibodies afterwards. For men who later choose to reverse their vasectomy, antisperm antibodies that have developed can interfere with conception. A "sperm allergy" can be reduced with use of immune balancing herbs like astragalus, reishi mushroom and cat's claw (an herbal anti-inflammatory). The Chinese combination Zhi bai du huang, which nourishes the kidney yin (the seat of reproductive health in Traditional Chinese Medicine), has had notably good results here. Zhi bai du huang is referred to in this country as Eight Flavor Rehmannia (containing the herbs prepared rehmannia, dogwood, Chinese yam, water plaintain, poria cocos, phellodendron, Anemarrhena asphodeloides) and is available in most natural foods stores.

What nutritional and lifestyle factors reduce female fertility?

Your over-the-counter medicine could be preventing conception. Research shows that overuse of NSAIDs (Non-steroidal anti-inflammatory drugs) like ibuprofen can induce "luteinized unruptured follicle syndrome," in which eggs are never released for conception. In fact, some "infertile" women have been able to complete successful pregnancies simply by stopping NSAID use!

Nutrient deficiencies like zinc, vitamin A, C and E also affect female reproductive health and block conception efforts. Being underweight, participating in excessive exercise like competitive marathons, or having severe anemia reduces female fertility by stopping menstruation. Smoking, excess alcohol or drugs can damage a woman's egg supply, hinder conception and lead to serious birth defects if pregnancy is achieved. Chronic emotional stress and depression reduce chances of successful pregnancy, too.

Excessive fiber intake or overuse of antibiotics can drastically reduce intestinal flora needed for estrogen circulation, and, therefore, reduce female fertility. Eating fish from contaminated waters may also decrease fertility. In one study, women who ate more than one fish meal per month of fish caught in Lake Ontario, known for its PCB contamination, took longer to get pregnant than other women.

Preliminary research from the *American Journal of Epidemiology* implicates milk consumption in women's infertility. Some women have trouble metabolizing the milk sugar, galactose; research shows older women with this problem may have a particularly hard time conceiving. Too much caffeine may decrease fertility, too. A recent large study found that women who consumed 300 mg of caffeine (equal to 2 or 3 cups of coffee) or more a day took longer to conceive than those who got less or none.

The Threat of Environmental Estrogen

Environmental hormones are so commonplace in modern society that there is no way to completely avoid them. They come from pollutants, drugs, hormone-injected meats and dairy foods, plastics, pesticides, and hormone replacement drugs for both sexes. Only in the last ten years has anyone realized how common environmental estrogens are in today's world. Nearly 40% of the pesticides used in commercial agriculture are suspected hormone disrupters. All of the Earth's waterways are connected, so chemical pollutants containing environmental hormones reach your food supply wherever you live. In 1996 the ENVIRONMENTAL PROTECTION AGENCY began implementing a congressionally mandated plan through EDSTAC (ENDOCRINE DISRUPTER SCREENING AND TESTING ADVISORY COMMITTEE) to test 87,000 compounds to determine their effect on the reproductive systems of humans and animals. However, due to the enormous scope of the project, a lack of funding and strong opposition from the chemical industry, progress is very slow moving.

Environmental estrogens can wreak havoc on male and female fertility. New research implicates hormone mimics from pollutants, estrogen exposure in the womb, chemical residues in food, water and plastics to infertility in both sexes. Multiple exposures to environmental estrogens disrupt conception efforts for both partners, affecting ovulation, and lowering sperm count and viability. Environmental estrogens seem to be implicated in most reproductive disorders like reproductive cancers, undescended testes, breast and uterine fibroids, polycystic ovarian syndrome, endometriosis, and pelvic inflammatory disease.

Estrogen-mimicking pollutants may, in fact, be changing the face of evolution. New reports show the effect of hormone disrupting pollutants on both wildlife and human health. Pallid sturgeons, found only in the Mississippi river, are now on the endangered species list as decades of exposure to pollutant PCBs (polychlorinated biphenyls) and DDT (dichloro-diphenyl-trichloroethane) have resulted in no new species birth for more than 10 years. Studies on turtles at the UNIVERSITY OF TEXAS find that even when environmental factors (like heat) are controlled to determine a male outcome, females or intersex turtles are hatched when even a small amount of PCBs are painted on the eggs. Exposure to PCBs has been linked to low sperm count for men, too. The newest research shows Atrazine, a weed killer, causes wildlife to develop the wrong sex organs. Atrazine use is so commonplace that it contaminates the water in states where it isn't even used.

Hormone disrupters can affect your entire endocrine system, including the system of your glands, hormones and cellular receptors in your body. They alter the production and breakdown of your own hormones, and the function of your hormone receptors — disrupting hormone balance at its developmental core. They can compete for hormone receptor sites in the body and bind to them in place of natural hormones, causing fluctuations in your hormonal levels. They are a serious concern for women in early pregnancy because a developing embryo is highly sensitive to estrogen disrupter toxicity. Some early research suggested these chemicals increase in potency when they're combined inside your body from several different sources, like from hormone-injected meats and pesticide-sprayed produce. However, new research has not duplicated these findings.

Are hormone disrupters impacting you? Signs that you may have estrogen disruption:

- **Breast inflammation and pain** that worsens before menstrual periods, usually followed by heavy, painful periods.
- **Weight gain:** especially in the hips.
- **Head hair loss and facial hair growth.**
- **Hot flashes:** a sign of hormone disruption in the brain.
- **Endometriosis:** now linked to dioxin, an air-born hormone disrupter.
- **Breast and uterine fibroid development, ovarian cysts, and pelvic inflammatory disease.**
- **Breast, uterine and reproductive organ cancer:** up to 60% more DDE, DDT and PCBs, known estrogen disrupters, in women with breast cancer.
- **Early puberty:** nearly half of African-American girls and 15% of Caucasian girls now begin to develop sexually by age 8, a clear indicator of estrogen disruption.

Are you at risk of exposure to estrogen disrupters? You may be especially exposed if:

1. You live in a high agricultural area; you eat a high fat diet (fatty areas of your body store pesticides and other agricultural chemicals)
2. You eat hormone-injected dairy foods or meats regularly.
3. You're on prescription HRT drugs or birth control pills.

With fertility blockers hitting us from every direction, what can hopeful parents do to improve their conception efforts? Is there any way to reduce your exposure to environmental estrogens and toxins from the environment?

First, cut back on fat and choose organic foods! Hormone disrupters accumulate in body fat... the reason a high fat diet is a major risk factor for long term exposure to them, and why it may lead to increased risk for hormone-driven cancers. The most recent testing shows at least 200 industrial and consumer product chemicals are present in the umbilical cords of U.S. children. An organic foods diet can protect your unborn child from this deluge of chemicals so present in today's environment.

Second, eat sea veggies like wakame, nori and dulse regularly. Algin, a gel like substance in sea greens, protects against chemical overload (often involved in breast cancer) by binding to chemical wastes so they can be eliminated safely from the body. Eat cruciferous veggies regularly to improve estrogen metabolism.

Third, avoid hormone-injected commercial meats, like beef. Choose hormone-free dairy products, too.

Fourth, use hormone-disrupting drugs like HRT drugs for menopause, and birth control pills only when all other options have been ruled out. Avoid hormone-mimics in personal care products, like placenta-containing hair rinses and conditioning treatments.

Chapter Two

Enhancing fertility, naturally

D iet is a critical key to successful conception… for both partners. I've seen over and over again that a good diet and lifestyle is critical for at least six months before trying to conceive for both partners. Nature tries in every way possible to ensure the survival of a new life, but the poor nutrition and stress of today's culture seems to be at the root of most fertility problems.

Guidelines for Male Fertility:

A "virility nutrition" program for men includes a short cleansing diet (see pg. 60-61 of this book for my 24-hour cleanse, it's a great cleanse for men to follow, too!). Then, focus on zinc-rich foods like pumpkin seeds, shellfish and seafood, protein rich foods, minimal sweets and dairy foods, and plenty of whole grains. Organic foods are important. A study in Lancet shows men who eat organic foods produce 43% more sperm than those who don't!

Healthy fats form a critical part of sperm cell membranes. Eating more foods rich in essential fatty acids like fish, flax seed, and borage seed can improve sperm quality and function. Unless you're very overweight, a weight loss diet may not be a good idea during preconception. Severe food limitation has a direct impact on the testicles. A study coming from MASSACHUSETTS GENERAL HOSPITAL shows that men's testosterone levels fall by 1/3 after fasting for 6-7 days. A man's fertility rise may take place in as little as 2 months after his diet improves. Do not smoke; avoid secondary smoke. Avoid areas with smog and pollutants.

Step-by-Step Fertility Diet for Men

You can follow a diet like this for 1–6 months. Add variety by including your choice of fresh, seasonal organic produce whenever possible. Choose free range meats and seafood from uncontaminated waters as much as possible. Note: Pesticide residues on commercially grown foods can disrupt male fertility by lowering sperm count. Buy organic!

On rising: Have a protein drink like METABOLIC RESPONSE MODIFIERS WHEY PUMPED or PURE FORM WHEY PROTEIN drink. Add 1–2 tsp. of HERBS AMERICA MACA MAGIC powder for extra fertility help.

Breakfast: Have whole grain cereal with apple or cranberry juice, or whole grain muffins with yogurt and fresh fruit, especially apples; or have poached or soft boiled eggs, and whole grain toast or couscous. Have a glass of fresh squeezed orange, tangerine or pomegranate juice for antioxidants.

Midmorning: Make a mix of nutritional yeast, bee pollen granules, wheat germ and oat bran: blend 2 tsp. into a superfood drink like GREEN FOODS GREEN MAGMA, WAKUNAGA KYO GREEN or ALOE LIFE DAILY GREENS. Or, have some low fat cottage cheese with nuts and seeds and whole grain crackers.

Lunch: Have a green leafy salad with a lemon oil or Italian dressing. Include celery, avocados and some grilled fresh fish like wild salmon if available. Or, have a hearty but low fat black beans and rice meal; or a roast turkey and spinach sandwich with a cup of lentil soup. Now is a good time to take your fertility enhancing supplements.

Mid-Afternoon: Have a cup of ginseng or licorice root tea (avoid licorice if you have high blood pressure) and a handful of pumpkin seeds for zinc.

Dinner: Have an Italian meal with whole grain or vegetable pasta, a light shellfish sauce and a green salad. Or, have a seafood and shellfish stew with steamed vegetables. Or have baked chicken or salmon with brown rice and peas.

Before bed: Have a nutritional yeast broth or small bottle of mineral water.

The male system responds quickly to nutritional changes. In addition, supplementation can produce dramatic renewed fertility results for men. Consider the following supplements for a man's fertility and virility program.

Supplement Choices for Men's Fertility

Choose 2 or 3 supplement recommendations. For detailed information on how herbs work for fertility, see pg. 42-47 of this book.

- **Natural vitamin E,** 400IU daily. New studies show vitamin E fights free radical damage and significantly improves sperm motility and fertility in men. A selenium supplement can improve sperm function. Try Vitamin E 400IU with selenium 200mcg daily (tests show pregnancies rise 21%).

- **Folic acid,** 800mcg daily (a key fertility nutrient for men, too) with **Zinc** 50–75mg daily or ETHICAL NUTRIENTS ZINC STATUS (tests for deficiency, too). A 2002 study published in *Fertility and Sterility* showed men who took folic acid and zinc together had a 74% increase in total sperm count.

- **B12** helps about half of men with low sperm count.

- Tests show the amino acid **L-carnitine,** 500–3000mg daily, boosts sperm quality in subfertile men.

- **L-arginine,** 2000–4000mg can raise sperm count and motility (contraindicated if you have herpes).

- **Pycnogenol** shows good results for sperm quality. In a clinical test with subfertile men, 200mg daily of pycnogenol improved sperm quality and motility by 38%.

- **Vitamin C,** 3000mg daily and **niacin** 500mg (good results for low sperm count or sperm clumping).

Men's fertility nutrient boosters:

SOLARAY MALE CAPS WITH ORCHIC EXTRACT, or COUNTRY LIFE MAX FOR MEN WITH RAW ORCHIC GLANDULAR. Try the carotene Lycopene (excellent results); CoQ10 60mg to enhance sperm energy production, as well as sperm count and motility.

Effective ginseng boosters: CRYSTAL STAR MALE PERFORMANCE™ caps or ginseng/damiana, 4 caps daily. To boost sperm quality and amount, try Siberian eleuthero extract (increases almost 30%); or LANE LABS FERTILE MALE (clinically shown to promote sperm count and mobility, good fertility results for our tester).

To remove heavy metals, especially lead from pesticides, consider CRYSTAL STAR TOXIN DETOX™ caps, 6 daily. Add extra glutathione for antioxidant defense. I like CARLSON GLUTATHIONE BOOSTER.

Guidelines for Female Fertility

A "fertility nutrition" program for a woman includes plenty of salads and greens, very low sugars, and a smaller volume of whole grains and nuts. Her diet should be low in saturated fats and trans fatty acids, moderate in Omega 6's from vegetable oils, but rich in essential fatty acids from sea greens and Omega-3 oils. We recommend fish and seafoods during pre-conception and after conception, rather than meat, (unless certified organic, because much of America's meat and poultry is antibiotic or hormone laced). A British study reveals women who eat more Omega 3 fatty acid rich fish during their last trimester give birth to bigger babies, who are less prone to problems like high blood pressure later in life. Newer research shows supplementing with omega 3 fatty acids may help prevent preeclampsia, postpartum depression, and a score of other problems like osteoporosis and breast cancer. HEALTH FROM THE SUN and BARLEANS ORGANIC OIL both make high quality Omega 3 fatty acid supplements that we've used with good results.

Limit dairy foods before conception. Too much dairy clogs the female system. Avoid refined carbs and sugar that feed candida yeast and imbalance androgen production. Imbalanced testosterone levels can lead to problems with embryonic development. Yeast infections and UTI's create an over-acidic environment which is inhospitable to sperm. Women with highly acidic vaginal pH may have difficulty becoming pregnant. (Esteemed colleague, Wayne Diamond, N.D. has used dandelion root tea in these cases with good results.) Excess sugar and alcohol can also interfere with estrogen metabolism. Cruciferous veggies like steamed broccoli and cauliflower help flush excess estrogens out. Foods with vitamin E like wheat germ, seeds, nuts and vegetable oils offer more body moisture. Magnesium-rich foods, like almonds, green leafy vegetables, avocado, carrots, citrus fruits, lentils, salmon counteract stress reactions that reduce fertility. Drink a cup of green tea every morning.

Important: Normalize your body weight before conception. Being overweight magnifies pregnancy problems like back and knee pain. Overweight women also increase their risk of developing toxemia or high blood pressure during pregnancy. On the other hand, severely underweight women may risk premature births or low birth weight babies. A woman's fertility rise may take 6–18 months after her diet change.

Step-by-Step Fertility Diet for Women

You can follow a diet like this for 1–6 months. Add more variety by including your choice of fresh, seasonal organic produce whenever possible. Choose free range meats and seafood from uncontaminated waters as much as possible. **Note:** Pesticide residues on commercially grown foods can disrupt conception efforts and possibly affect the future hormonal health of a developing child.

On rising: Have a cup of green tea every morning. Add 1 tsp. of royal jelly or one vial PRINCE OF PEACE RED GINSENG ROYAL JELLY for extra fertility help.

Breakfast: Have some fresh fruit mixed into low fat yogurt; or have my personal breakfast of champions: brown rice, with steamed cruciferous vegetables, sprinkled sea vegetables and a little tamari sauce and fresh ginger.

Midmorning: Have fresh carrot juice, red clover infusion (see pg. 43) or CRYSTAL STAR CONCEPTIONS™ TEA (highly recommended) with 1 tsp. BARLEANS HIGH LIGNAN FLAX SEED OIL (Omega 3's). If you're still hungry, have some crunchy vegetables and a veggie dip.

Lunch: Have a turkey, avocado and baby greens sandwich or salad; or a seafood and veggie pasta salad; or a light oriental soup and salad, with sea veggies and rice crackers.

Midafternoon: Have another cup of red clover infusion, red raspberry tea or CRYSTAL STAR CONCEPTIONS™ TEA (highly recommended).

Dinner: have a Chinese stir fry with dark greens and mushrooms, and miso soup with sea greens chopped on top. Or, have baked or poached seafood with steamed cruciferous vegetables and brown rice or couscous; or a vegetarian quiche with whole grain crust and small salad.

Before bed: have a glass of mineral water, or a relaxing herb tea like chamomile tea or CRYSTAL STAR STRESS ARREST™ TEA.

Supplement Choices for Women's Fertility

Women's bodies respond well to gentle whole herb remedies for infertility problems rather than many high potency supplements. Remember, B vitamins are a critical part of women's reproductive health and minerals like calcium should be in ample supply as needs increase during pregnancy.

Choose 2-3 recommendations. For detailed information on how herbs work for fertility, see pg. 42-47 of this book.

Preconception (normalize menstrual cycle):

- **Vitex extract** promotes ovulation and helps correct luteal phase defect; using vitamin C 750mg daily helps promote ovulation in women with luteal phase defect.

- **Balance hormones:** Crystal Star Female Harmony™ caps 4 daily with Evening Primrose Oil for EFAs, 4 daily; or Crystal Star Pro-Est Balance™ roll-on or Moon Maid Pro-meno Wild Yam cream for 1 month with extra B6 to reduce chance of miscarriage. Pure Essence Labs Fem Creme natural progesterone cream helps avoid miscarriage caused by luteal phase failure. For more on reducing miscarriage risk, see pg. 66 of this book.

- **Increase libido to maximize conception potential:** High Potency Royal Jelly 2 tsp. daily- try Prince of Peace Red Ginseng, Royal Jelly vials; Aromatherapy rose oil; or Histidine 1000mg daily for more sexual enjoyment. Red raspberry tea helps tone uterus (excellent results). Licorice extract helps hormone balance for polycystic ovary syndrome.

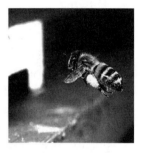

- **Women's fertility nutrient boosters:** red clover infusion; Crystal Star Conceptions™ tea, (add ashwagandha extract drops); Herbs America Maca Magic caps for a fertility and libido lift (highly recommended); Crystal Star Ocean Minerals™ caps (iodine, potassium, silica from sea veggies) to guard against birth defects. Consider a multivitamin-mineral supplement for women's fertility like Fairhaven Health FertilAid for women. Vitamin E 400IU 2x daily; B-complex, like Nature's Secret Ultimate B with extra B6 100mg, PABA 400mg (75% effective in 1 small trial) and folic acid 800mcg daily. Country life sublingual B-12, 2500mcg daily. Lane Labs Advacal Ultra with magnesium (highly recommended). Cayenne-ginger caps, motherwort tea, hawthorn extract 4x daily for a feeling of well-being.

- **Protease enzymes,** like Crystal Star Dr. Enzyme™ with Protease & Bromelain or Transformation Purezyme caps, taken between meals keep fibroid growths in check and cleanse toxins in the bloodstream. See ovarian cysts, fibroids and endometriosis pages in this book for more information on how to overcome these problems for healthy conception.

Important fertility guidelines for both sexes: Avoid or reduce consumption of tobacco, caffeine, and alcohol. (Moderate wine is ok until conception.) Take care to keep your personal environment free of toxins. Living near toxic landfills increases risk for DNA abnormalities like Down syndrome. Both men and women should limit their saturated fat intake to about 10% of the diet. Especially reduce sugary foods (artificial sweeteners like aspartame are particularly hazardous for your unborn child) and meats that are regularly laced with nitrates and-or hormones, like red meats, and smoked, cured and processed meats. Much of the research we're seeing today shows a high intake of antioxidants sets a good stage for fertility. Vitamin C, in particular, is an important fertility nutrient for men and women. Semen contains high levels of vitamin C. Low levels of vitamin C contribute to the death of the corpus luteum (a mature ovarian follicle that ruptures to release a potentially mature egg) in research animals. Both sexes should be sure to eat plenty of vitamin C rich foods like citrus fruits, papaya, kiwi, potatoes, cauliflower and broccoli to help overcome nutrient deficiency based infertility. Zinc is an important fertility nutrient for both sexes. Zinc is important to synthesis of DNA and RNA. Zinc supplements have been shown to improve fertility in women. Zinc deficiency is also linked to men's infertility. Incorporate these zinc-rich foods in your diet: nuts, seeds, high quality seafood and shellfish, nutritional yeast, and eggs.

> It's easy for couples dealing with infertility problems to lose their spark while focusing on the mechanics of conception.
>
> Enjoy and be patient with each other on this journey.
>
> Try to handle disappointments and setbacks with love and compassion.

Bodywork and Relaxation Therapies

Bodywork therapies are an integral part of natural healing's success for infertility. Therapies like acupuncture and massage have documented success for many types of infertility and are a viable choice for reproductive health. Here are a few examples of bodywork therapies you can start using today to improve your fertility status.

Exercise recharges the cardiovascular system and boosts testosterone and sperm production. In one study, 78 healthy, but sedentary men were studied during nine months of regular exercise. The men exercised for 60 minutes a day, three days a week. Every man in the study reported significantly enhanced sexuality, including increased frequency, performance and satisfaction. The rise in sexuality was even correlated with how much each man's fitness improved!

Exercise is also a great way to keep body fat down, another conception inhibitor. Body fat levels just 10-15% above normal can disrupt fertility efforts for both partners. I think exercising together is a great way for couples experiencing fertility problems to enhance their sex life. Get light exercise, and morning sunshine every day possible. Deep breathing exercises, especially during long walks together, are very beneficial. But don't get too carried away, excessive exercise can disrupt fertility efforts for both sexes.

Deep tissue massage

Deep tissue massage can help clear blocked fallopian tubes and increase pregnancy chances. Female infertility is routinely caused by pelvic adhesions, blocked tubes or other types of trauma or inflammation in the reproductive organs. While long believed that surgery procedures were the only way to even partially decrease these problems, bodywork therapists have found deep tissue work can not only decrease mechanical blockages, but also reduce pelvic pain and improve sexual arousal and orgasm for women. What a bonus!

In a preliminary study conducted by *Clear Passages* in Florida, of 8 infertile women treated with deep tissue massage, 50% gave birth to healthy, full term babies. (Current fertility technologies offer about 20%-40% success rate.) Subsequent studies show even better outcomes, with up to 70% of patients becoming pregnant naturally within 1 year. More good news: WURN Treatment is more affordable than IVF, at about $3500 for a course, and is more likely to be covered by insurance. The WURN technique can also improve your chances of conception if you're planning to do IVF. Larry and Belinda Wurn, the husband-wife team running *Clear Passages,* have their research published on *Medscape General Medicine, Ob/ Gyn & Women's Health* on the web for couples wanting more information. Also, check out *www.clearpassage.com.*

39

The Amazing Role of Acupuncture

Try acupuncture if you are considering IVF. Acupuncture has a centuries long history of safety and effectiveness, and it may help you get pregnant faster if you're using IVF. In China, where IVF is not common, acupuncture and herbal remedies are the first choice for infertility problems. A handful of studies from the U.S. and Europe reveal that acupuncture enhances the success rates of IVF treatments. Tests show receiving acupuncture 30 minutes before and after IVF increases chances of successful embryo implantation and reduces the chance of miscarriage. The best results are achieved when treatments are received once a week during the month or two leading up to your treatment, and then continued once or twice a week through the whole cycle.

How does acupuncture work for fertility?

Most practitioners of Chinese medicine view infertility as a weakness of qi (vital energy) in the liver and kidneys. Acupuncturists insert tiny needles into various points on the body meridians to help normalize the flow of qi. Acupuncture helps release stagnancy patterns or obstructions in the body, and reduce anxiety that may be preventing conception. Infertility caused by poor blood flow to the uterus can be greatly improved through acupuncture treatments. Acupuncture also increases circulation to the ovaries, allowing for healthier eggs, and to the uterus, strengthening the lining so it will be able to carry a pregnancy to full term. There are many reports of acupuncture improving sperm count, motility and morphology (shape) for infertile or subfertile men. In one 1987 study reported in the *Journal of Chinese Acupuncture*, of 248 men who received acupuncture to treat infertility, 89 were cured, 77 made significant improvements and 85 experienced no change. Other studies show similar positive results for men. Using meditation with fertility treatments may also yield good results.

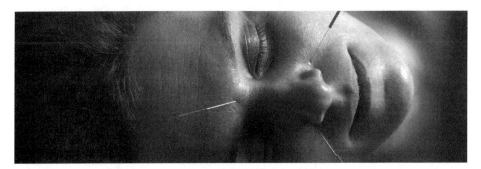

The Mind Body Connection

Scientific evidence is piling up showing the mind-body connection is important for conception, even for women who use fertility drugs. A study published in *Fertility and Sterility* found women who expressed negative emotions at the beginning of IVF treatment were 93% less likely to have a baby than those who expressed positive feelings. In another study funded by the NATIONAL INSTITUTE OF MENTAL HEALTH, over half of couples with fertility problems gave birth one year after joining a mind-body program, compared to 20% in the control group. Alice Domar, author of *Healing Mind, Healthy Woman*, documents a 55% success rate for women using relaxation techniques to help them get pregnant, compared to a 20% success rate for women who used only medical fertility technologies.

Women who feel undeserving of having a child or who have chronic intense stress, guilt or other emotional issues also may have a tougher time getting pregnant. Anxiety, depression and feeling of inadequacy about infertility only compounds the problem. In these cases, make a conscious effort to clean up the emotional clutter to clear your fertility pathways for your own future and that of your child. Sessions with skilled practitioner of guided imagery or family therapist can produce good results. Prayer, meditation, keeping a journal and relaxation techniques like deep breathing can also reduce stress that may be decreasing fertility.

Having said that, our burgeoning population shows that many "stressed out" women can and do get pregnant all the time. Still, for women who are having difficulty getting pregnant reducing stress can make all the difference. Some women are just too overworked to conceive. Women with infertility issues who are working 60-80 hours a week might want to look at their inability to conceive as a sign from their bodies that they need to take time out from their jobs to nurture themselves. And women who are already pregnant or planning to get pregnant need to make a conscious decision to put their mind-body health first for their own sake and that of their child. A new study in the journal *Child Development* shows that high stress during pregnancy increases a child's susceptibility to ADHD later in life.

A highly nutritious diet and relaxation therapies can make all the difference for couples experiencing fertility difficulties. Whole herbs are another good choice with profound effects for enhanced fertility and sexuality.

Fertility Enhancing Herbs

Whole herbs address a multitude of infertility causes: hormone imbalance; body toxicity; stress; female obstructions and scarring. While herbal medicines have been used safely for preconception needs for thousands of years, some herbs should never be used during pregnancy because they are too strong for a fetus or they can stimulate uterine contractions. For a complete list of herbs to avoid during pregnancy, see pg.106.

Herbs can help a man overcome low sperm count or declining fertility, even sexual performance problems. Herbs are an especially good choice for older men wanting to sustain virility, energy and potency during andropause.

Women's Whole Herb Choices

Black cohosh and blue cohosh (*Cimicifuga spp.*) are toning herbs for female imbalances like prolapsed uterus and fibroids. CRYSTAL STAR WOMEN'S BEST FRIEND™ with black cohosh can help the body normalize from prolapses or fibroids, but should not be used during pregnancy. See pg. 57 for details on herbal formulas for fibroids and endometriosis. Black and blue cohosh are also sometimes used to aid in childbirth, but I only suggest this under the guidance of a clinical herbalist with experience in midwifery.

Dong quai (*Angelica sinensis*), used extensively in Traditional Chinese Medicine for female complaints, helps to regulate ovulation, menstruation and can tone a weak uterus. Dong quai is particularly helpful for women stopping oral contraceptive use. As an herbal source of vitamin B12 and folic acid, dong quai can help treat infertility secondary to anemia. Note: Dong quai can promote menstrual flow in some women. In many cases, this is a good thing, clearing blood stagnation that affects fertility. (From a TCM perspective, stagnant blood is a major cause of infertility in women.) This is normally a temporary reaction and a sign that the body is normalizing. Having a cup or two of nettles tea can help curtail heavy flow. For the best results, seek guidance from a professional herbalist trained in TCM. I myself use only whole dong quai in herbal combinations, like CRYSTAL STAR CONCEPTIONS™ TEA, which is well tolerated by women for their self-care. Avoid using dong quai with blood-thinning medications.

Green tea (*Camellia sinensis*) tastes great, is widely available and it may increase your chances of getting pregnant. Research on green tea already shows good results for conception. A study from the *American Journal of Public Health* shows drinking just 1/2 cup or more of green tea daily can double the odds of conception during one cycle. As an antioxidant, green tea may help repair free radical damage linked to infertility problems in men and women. Don't overdo it though. Just 1–2 cups a day is fine. Excess caffeine from tea can decrease fertility.

False Unicorn (*Chamalerium luteum*) has been used for centuries as a fertility aid. Specifically, it is a uterine tonic that decreases pelvic congestion. Clinical herbalists use false unicorn to help prevent miscarriage caused by uterine weakness. False unicorn can also be used to regulate menstruation and to strengthen the uterine lining. Dosage: 5–30 drops of extract daily. During pregnancy, use false unicorn only in the last few weeks to prepare for labor, or with advice from a clinical herbalist.

Licorice root (*Glycrrhiza glabra*), used in Chinese herbal formulas to harmonize the activity of individual herbs, is a menstruation regulator with anti-inflammatory properties. It offers balancing activity for estrogen and testosterone levels, and specifically benefits women with infertility related to Polycystic Ovary Syndrome. Licorice root works well in an extract. Try 1-1.5 tsp. 3x daily. (Contraindicated if you have high blood pressure).

Red clover (*Trifolium pratense*) is best known today as a hormonal balancer for menopausal women, but it can also be used to promote fertility. Red clover is rich in plant estrogens which can promote fertility in women with estrogen deficiency. Wise Woman Susun Weed reports conception enhancing results for women who drink up to 1-4 cups a day of a strong red clover blossoms infusion. Weed's recipe? She adds 1 oz. by weight of dried red clover blossoms to a quart sized canning jar, fills the jar with boiling water, screws on a lid and lets the mixture sit overnight or for at least four hours. For improved palatability, she adds a teaspoon or two of peppermint leaves. Weed explains the dried blossoms are especially helpful for women with scarring of the fallopian tubes, irregular menstrual cycle or "unexplained" infertility.

A **red raspberry** (*Rubus idaeus*) tea combination: Herbal teas, the gentlest of all herbal mediums, can maximize your conception efforts. Crystal Star Conceptions™ tea is a broad spectrum formula that helps maximize conception potential without the side effects or risk of fertility drugs. Red raspberry has a long history of safe and effective use as a natural fertility enhancer, and is included as a nutritive, astringent herb that helps prepare the uterus for healthy conception. Sea greens and whole herbs in the blend are loaded with B vitamins, EFAs, and critical minerals like calcium, silica, magnesium and iodine to shore up nutrient supply and establish a body environment favorable for conception. For best results, take Conceptions™ tea for 3 to 4 months prior to conception while following a "fertility nutrition" program for women. Adding Ashwagandha drops to the tea can give it an extra "fertility boost." Ashwagandha, the great Ayurveda tonic (especially for sexual energy) has been successfully used to treat female infertility for many years.

Squaw vine: Native Americans used squaw vine (*Mitchella repens*) as a fertility tonic for women. It can also be helpful during the last trimester of pregnancy to strengthen the uterine muscles and facilitate child birth. Interestingly, squaw vine both improves uterine tone and relaxes spasms. See pg. 105 for information on squaw vine's use during late pregnancy.

Tribulus terrestris (Puncture vine), an herb native to India and Africa increases sex drive without the side effects of traditional hormone drugs like weight gain (estrogen) or masculinization (testosterone). In one study, 2/3 of women treated with tribulus report renewed sexual interest! There's also some evidence which suggests tribulus may help regulate ovulation. Dosage: Source Naturals Tribulus Terrestris is a good choice, 750-1500mg daily.

True unicorn (*Aletris farinosa*), a widely used digestive tonic by the Native American Catawba, is also a useful herb for uterine prolapse, irregular menstrual cycle, and threatened miscarriage. Use just 1/4 tsp. of powdered root for one cup of tea. Best under guidance from a clinical herbalist. Overdosage can cause diarrhea and vomiting.

Vitex extract (*Vitex agnus*), known as "chaste tree," was used in the days of the ancient Greeks to suppress libido. But modern research on vitex reveals it can help normalize ovulation for women with ovulatory disorders. It has specific benefits for improving a short luteal phase and Polycystic Ovary Syndrome. Vitex works by stimulating luteinizing hormone production and reducing release of follicle-stimulating hormone. It also supports pituitary gland health and encourages estrogen and progesterone balance in the body. A 1993 study from Hamburg reveals vitex also helps reduce high prolactin levels, linked to women's infertility. Two double-blind studies show vitex extract increases a woman's fertility and chances of successful conception. Dosage: Take 10-15 drops of the extract, 2–3 times a day for the first two weeks of your cycle.

Wild yam: Before synthetic hormones became widely available, whole wild yam (*Dioscorea villosa*) was used as the source material to make early contraceptive pills. Wild yam contains diosgenin, a saponin with hormone-like effects which can be converted to progesterone in a laboratory. While scientists have shown that diosgenin cannot convert into progesterone in the female body, my experience and that of many women I have worked with over the years shows me that wild yam offers mild progesterone balancing activity without the side effects of hormone drugs. Regarding fertility, its action is complex. In large doses (3000mg or more daily), wild yam has anti-fertility action, but in small doses (50 to 100mg), it can help promote conception. For fertility purposes, use whole wild yam in combinations like CONCEPTIONS™ TEA or use it only in the first half of the menstrual cycle (before ovulation).

Note: If you're worried by the 1999 studies from Loma Linda University linking herbs like St. John's wort, ginkgo biloba and echinacea to infertility, know that the herbs were only tested in a test tube on hamster eggs. It is highly improbable that the same herbs used in a living animal or human would have the same effect. Whole herbs, as gentle healing foods, are processed by our enzymatic systems… neutralizing, in the vast majority of cases, potential for toxicity.

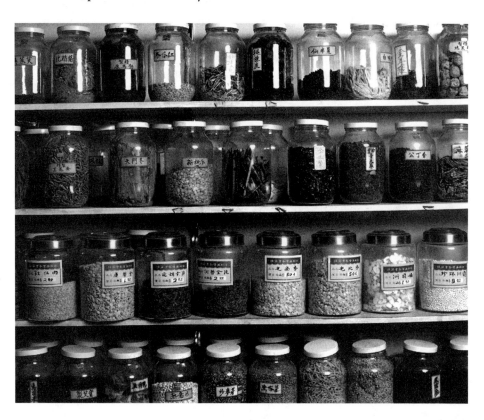

Men's Whole Herb Choices

Men experience a gradual decline in fertility as they age. Tests show men over 50 have 20% reduction in semen volume. Men at 30 have a 40% chance of abnormal sperm motility, men at 50 have an 80% chance. Still, advances in fertility technologies mean men who are producing any sperm at all have a very good chance of having a biological child. In addition, numerous plant medicines normalize sperm quantity and quality for healthy conception. Many herbs also enhance libido and sexual performance for men.

Damiana (*Turnera diffusa*), used by the Mayan people of Central America, is a useful libido promoter for both men and women trying to conceive. With mild testosterone-like effects, Damiana helps restore health to the reproductive organs and is especially beneficial for men who suffer from impotence or premature ejaculation. I recommend damiana in herbal combinations or by itself in capsules or in a tea. 300-600mg daily is a good dose.

Ginseng species nourish and tone the male reproductive system. Research published in the *Journal of Urology* shows red panax ginseng improves erectile function for impotent men. **Chinese ginseng** (*Panax g.*), has been shown to increase sperm count, improve sperm motility, decrease prolactin levels, and boost testosterone concentration. Animal tests reveal Siberian *eleuthero*, a ginseng-like plant from Russia, produces an almost 30% increase in semen production and a 50% drop in stillborn births. I recommend a ginseng-based combination like CRYSTAL STAR MALE PERFORMANCE™ CAPSULES. IMPERIAL ELIXIR, SUPERIOR TRADING and PRINCE OF PEACE also offer high-quality ginseng products.

Guizhi-Fuling-Wan: The Chinese combination Guizhi-Fuling-Wan (Cinnamon and Poria Formula) has been shown clinically to reduce infertility caused by varicocele. Test participants took 7.5 grams of the combination daily for at least 3 months. 80% of patients overcame their varicocele and there was a 71% increase in sperm concentration and 62% increase in sperm motility. In TCM, Guizhi-Fuling-Wan is used to improve circulation in the lower abdomen and decrease blood stagnation. Consider Plum Flowers Cinnamon & Poria teapills, available at natural foods stores.

Peruvian maca (*Lepidium meyenii*), often called "the herbal viagra," boosts sex drive and performance for older men. Maca is excellent as an endurance enhancer and can improve erectile dysfunction. Modern Maca research reveals animals with low testosterone given maca experience a significant improvement in sexual activity. Further, tests show taking 1500–3000mg of maca daily for 4 months can increase seminal volume, sperm count and sperm motility in men. LANE LABS FERTIL MALE with maca is clinically shown to promote sperm count and motility and we personally know of cases where it's been used with good results. HERBS AMERICA MACA MAGIC is another high quality maca product we've worked with.

Pygeum (*Pygeum africanum*) is used extensively in Europe for prostate enlargement. Research shows it balances prostatic fluid pH, and even improves the ability of sperm to survive outside the body. Pygeum is also helpful in cases of impotence. **Saw palmetto berries** (*Serenoa repens*), native to the U.S. and the West Indies, are clinically shown to reduce prostate swelling and related symptoms, like difficult or frequent urination. Saw palmetto is also a primary tissue builder and gland stimulating herb for toning the male reproductive system. Saw palmetto and pygeum are combined in CRYSTAL STAR PROSTATE PROTECTOR™capsules.

Ayurvedic **tribulus terrestris**, strengthens the reproductive system for men and women. It is proven to improve both low sperm count and poor sperm motility. Additionally, research shows tribulus can improve sexual desire and activity in cases of prostatitis, shrunken testes, and syndromes involving undescended testes. It even increases sperm motility and ejaculate quality in men after surgery for a varicocele (varicose vein within spermatic cord), another common cause of male infertility. The researchers used dosages of 1500mg for 60-90 days. SOURCE NATURALS TRIBULUS TERRESTRIS is a good brand to try.

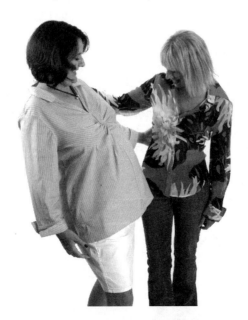

Chapter Three

Overcoming sexually transmitted disease & reproductive blockages

Sexually transmitted diseases (STDs) are widespread, reaching epidemic proportions in most places in the world. It is estimated that one out of every five Americans has an incurable sexually transmitted infection; 15 million new infections occur each year. STDs are a significant health threat at every level of American life. No treatment for impotence, no questions about infertility, no decision about conception can be made without considering the STD quotient. Genital warts, herpes, gonorrhea and chlamydia rates are rising fast, particularly among women. At this writing, over 36 million people worldwide are living with HIV or AIDS, a life threatening STD. The consequences for fertility and childbirth can be devastating.

STD Prevention & Treatment

Most STDs are extremely contagious. Even though precautions may be taken during active stages when an STD is recognized, many like herpes and HPV (human papilloma virus) can be transmitted during inactive stages. Because a great number of people are asymptomatic after they are infected, STDs may be unknowingly spread for years, causing reproductive damage. Women are in greater danger then men. Anatomically, women are more vulnerable to STDs than men, because a man's infected secretions remain in the woman's vagina after intercourse.

A monogamous relationship with an uninfected partner and/or abstinence are your best protection against STDs. If that is not possible, proper use of the male condom and abstinence during STD outbreaks can decrease your risk of contracting an infection. Female-controlled prevention technology is not yet on a par with the male condom. Female condoms are still extraordinarily clumsy.

Be very careful in your choice of sexual partners, sexual practices and STD protection methods. Sexual disease consequences are severe because they are frequently irreversible. The problem goes even beyond the woman herself. Her sexual responsibility may affect not only her ability to have a child, but through transmitted infection, her children's health. Because STDs are extremely contagious, they often affect both partners' ability to conceive, no matter who had the disease first.

Do you have an STD?

Check with your physician right away if you're having any of the following symptoms which may appear 2 to 3 weeks after sexual contact. Some STDs are treatable if caught early. You can greatly improve your chances of healthy conception by treating an STD early before major damage to the reproductive organs is done.

- Thick discharge in some men and all women; urethritis; pelvic pain; difficulty conceiving (chlamydia)
- Headache, stiff neck, fever, genital itch; genital blisters that swell, fester and rupture; shooting pains in thighs and legs (herpes)
- Itchy, unsightly warts in the genital or anal area (genital warts, a high risk factor for cervical cancer for women)
- Cloudy green or yellow discharge, painful urination, yeast infection, pelvic inflammation (gonorrhea)
- Severe itchiness, thin, foamy yellowish discharge with foul odor (trichomonas)

STDs Impact on Fertility & Childbirth

In men, STDs weaken sperm production, damage the testes, scar the vas deferens, reduce sexual vitality and cause a lingering low level infection that affects the entire immune system. There can be severe complications from STD's in women, too - like infertility and increased risk of cervical cancer and HIV. STDs damage the whole female reproductive area, often producing lingering infections, scarring and adhesions throughout the pelvic region which can prevent conception. 10–40% of women infected with gonorrhea or chlamydia will develop PID (pelvic inflammatory disease) leading to scarring in the fallopian tubes. Statistics from the Centers for Disease Control reveal that of women who develop PID, 20% will become infertile from tubal scarring; 9% will develop an ectopic pregnancy (potentially life threatening); and 18% will experience chronic pelvic pain.

STDs can lead to childbirth complications as they are passed to the infant in the birth canal. Herpes can cause chronic eye infections, blindness or even fatal infections. HPV (human papilloma virus) can cause life threatening warts on the vocal cords (Laryngeal papillomatosis). Laryngeal papillomatosis is a rare, but extremely serious, childbirth risk. Gonorrhea and chlamydia can also result in conjunctivitis and pneumonia in a newborn. HIV/AIDS is another life threatening infection that can be transmitted to an infant during child labor.

I strongly recommend routine prenatal STD screening to help reduce devastating infant infections. Always tell your doctor if you know you have a sexually transmitted infection. Today's doctors are increasingly understanding about these types of health problems. Preventive treatment, both medical and herbal, can help protect your unborn child.

Overcoming STDs: What are the best natural treatments for STDs?

For many years, the only treatment for sexually transmitted diseases was long courses of powerful, but immune-depressing drugs. Today, we are rediscovering the power of herbal remedies and other natural treatments against STDs. A strong arsenal of herbal remedies and supplements can fortify the body against both outbreaks and some of the devastating consequences.

Some STDs respond better to natural treatments than others. Those with acute symptoms may require a short initial course of antibiotic drugs to give the body a stabilizing boost. In the case of chlamydia, gonorrhea, trichomonas and syphilis, medical treatment with antibiotics is the preferred first treatment of choice, followed by an immune recovery diet with supportive supplements. A doctor who is knowledgeable about holistic methods can determine whether antibiotics or other drugs are necessary, or whether natural remedies alone will be effective. Even when conventional medicine is needed, adding natural therapies under the supervision of a qualified professional with alternative knowledge can greatly assist healing.

Note that unless specified, the STD remedies in this section are recommended for pre-conception needs. If you're already pregnant and have been diagnosed with, or suspect you may have a STD, I recommend you work with a holistic physician. Medical treatment can help protect you and your unborn child. Viral STD outbreaks like herpes can be reduced during pregnancy through stress reduction and a balanced, whole foods diet. However, if you're having an active herpes or genital warts outbreak during labor, a C-section will be necessary.

STD Recovery Diet

Diet is an essential component of recovery. Emphasis must be on optimal nutrient foods that can strengthen your body and build strong immune response. Reduce dietary fats, caffeine, sugar, and alcohol. Don't smoke. It seriously depresses immune response.

- Eat plenty of fresh vegetables, especially high chlorophyll, blood cleansing leafy greens. Have a salad every day with flax oil or olive oil dressing for essential fatty acids.
- Have a glass of fresh vegetable juice (any blend) daily.
- Eat only whole foods. No junk or heavily processed foods.
- Eat about 2 tablespoons of dried sea vegetables daily.
- Eat yogurt or other cultured foods for friendly flora.
- Add neutralizing superfoods for detoxification support: SUN CHLORELLA, 2 pkts. daily, CRYSTAL STAR RESTORE YOUR STRENGTH™; ALOE LIFE ALOE GOLD drink 1-2 tbsp. daily.
- Drink purified water, about eight 8-oz. glasses daily.

Some supplements and superfoods we work with to help build immune strength:

Use CRYSTAL STAR DETOX BLOOD PURIFIER™ capsules for one month as a blood cleanser (with red clover, licorice root, hawthorn, sea buckthorn, hawthorn, rose hips, burdock, pau d'arco, sarsaparilla, fo ti, alfalfa, buckthorn, echinacea, garlic, goldenseal, astragalus, kelp, dulse, American ginseng, bladderwrack, Oregon grape, poria cocus, yellow dock, prickly ash, dandelion, ginger, capsicum, milk thistle seed, Irish moss): followed by FIBER & HERBS COLON CLEANSE™ to rid the colon of re-infection (with butternut, triphala, cascara sagrada, turkey rhubarb, psyllium, fennel, slippery elm, barberry, licorice, ginger, Irish moss, capsicum).

Use enzyme therapy to help break down protein pathogen invaders in your blood supply so they can be destroyed by your immune system. A formula like CRYSTAL STAR DR. ENZYME WITH PROTEASE & BROMELAIN™ or PUREZYME from TRANSFORMATION ENZYME CORPORATION helps cleanse the bloodstream and address infectious viruses, pathogenic bacteria, funguses and parasites.

Olive Leaf Extract has been used with remarkable success against every infective organism type—viral, bacterial, fungal, and protozoan (parasitic) infections. New clinical experience shows that olive leaf extract is an effective treatment for an incredible list of serious modern health problems. Herpes I and II, human herpes virus 6 and 7, HIV virus, flu virus, the common cold, meningitis, Epstein-Barr Virus, encephalitis, shingles, chronic fatigue, hepatitis B, pneumonia, tuberculosis, gonorrhea, malaria, severe diarrhea, blood poisoning, and dental, ear, urinary tract and surgical infections all respond to olive leaf. Recent lab tests have found that olive leaf extract kills 56 pathogens. Amazing! I have worked with and highly recommend PROLIVE OLIVE LEAF EXTRACT by NUTRICOLOGY.

Eat fermented foods like yogurt or take protective acidophilus; UAS LABS DDS-PLUS, PURE ESSENCE FLOR-ALIVE, and JARROW JARRO-DOPHILUS, especially if you are taking a long course of antibiotics for an STD.

Detoxify your liver with MILK THISTLE SEED extract or CRYSTAL STAR LIVER CLEANSE FLUSHING TEA™.

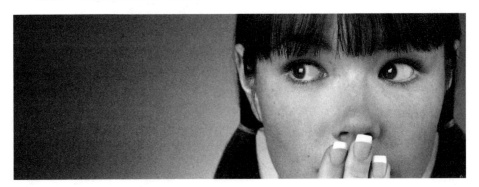

Take Vitamin C as an antioxidant and antiviral agent to stimulate immune function. An ascorbic acid flush often works well as part of a natural healing program for STDs.

Take antioxidants to neutralize free radicals, balance your body chemistry, strengthen immune response and protect your blood cells from damage. Here are some recommendations:

- CAROTENOID COMPLEX by COUNTRY LIFE
- ALPHA LIPOIC ACID—100 mg, twice daily by NOW FOODS
- GRAPEFRUIT SEED EXTRACT CAPS and skin spray—by NUTRIBIOTIC
- GERMANIUM by NUTRICOLOGY

Lifestyle-Bodywork Support Therapy

- Apply ice packs to lesions for pain and inflammation relief. Ice may also be applied as a preventive measure when the sufferer feels a flare-up coming on.
- Get some early morning sunlight on the sores every day for healing Vitamin D.
- Stress reduction techniques like biofeedback, meditation and imagery help prevent outbreaks.
- Acupuncture is effective for herpes.

Breakthrough Therapies and Products

The following section highlights a few of the best natural therapies for STDs we have experienced success with today. Complete natural healing programs for sexually transmitted diseases are available in the bestselling book, *Healthy Healing,* 12th Edition by this book's co-author, Linda Page, Ph.D., and traditional naturopath.

Genital Herpes (Simplex 2)

Genital herpes affects up to 45 million Americans, with almost 1 million new cases each year!

A low arginine diet: A diet containing significant amounts of arginine aggravates herpes. Foods to avoid include: chocolate; nuts like peanuts, almonds, cashews, walnuts; seeds like sunflower and sesame; and coconut. Foods containing a moderate amount of arginine should be eaten with discretion. These include wheat, soy, lentils, oats, corn, rice, barley, tomato, and squash. Avoid these foods until outbreak blisters have disappeared. Immune-suppressants like caffeine, alcohol, and tobacco should also be eliminated from your diet.

Lysine compounds are a key. Here's why: The herpes virus needs arginine to reproduce. Both amino acids, lysine and arginine look similar to the virus. Lysine therapy fools the virus into thinking it is arginine, and the virus will take lysine, if it is available instead, thus blocking virus development, and keeping it from reactivating.

Red marine algae (Dumonticaea, Gigartina species) can actively affect several herpes types (HSV-I, HSV-II, EBV and Zoster). It works well topically as well as internally. Red algae affects herpes virus in a variety of ways:

- Inhibits DNA and RNA formation of the virus.

- Works as a selective immune stimulant which prevents the proliferation of suppressor T-cells, thus allowing the immune system to control the recurrence of herpes episodes.

- Alters the biochemistry of the body (creating an alkaline condition) that causes an unsuitable environment for the herpes virus to proliferate, and allows the body to rebuild healthy tissue.

For ongoing outbreak prevention, consider a formula with both L-lysine and red marine algae like CRYSTAL STAR HERPEX™ capsules. Both HERPEX™ capsules and topical gel can be used to help reduce outbreak severity and also as a protective measure. DIAMOND FORMULAS HERPANACINE capsules are another trusted favorite we've worked with.

If you're already pregnant and have herpes: CRYSTAL STAR HERPEX™ topical lysine gel can also be used safely to support recovery as directed. Use with echinacea/burdock root tea, 2 cups daily to strengthen immune defenses and purify the blood. Let steep for an hour or so for potency. DIAMOND FORMULAS HERPANACINE caps, 4 daily, are another good choice for supporting immune recovery during pregnancy.

MERIX HEALTH PRODUCTS RELEEV capsules and ointment also offer excellent anti-viral activity (highly recommended).

Genital Warts - HPV (Human Papillomavirus) - Cervical Dysplasia

HPV affects 20 million people in the United States. 5.5 million more are infected every year. In fact, HPV infects more people every year than any other sexually transmitted disease (STD).

Add folic acid foods like lima beans, whole wheat and nutritional yeast as protection against cervical dysplasia. Include extra vitamin B complex 100 mg daily.

Usnea extract helps deal with the virus. Dosage: 30-40 drops, 3-5 times per day until symptoms improve. For 1 month, give your body an ascorbic acid flush with 1/4 tsp. vitamin C powder with bioflavonoids every hour until the stool turns loose. Then take vitamin C 5000mg with bioflavonoids daily for a month.

For acute viral wart outbreaks, try WELL IN HAND WART WONDER topical treatment (highly recommended). Or make up goldenseal/chaparral vaginal suppositories (powders mixed with vitamin A oil). They are extremely helpful for women with venereal warts or dysplasia, rendering many symptom-free.

An herbal vag pack can detox the vaginal area. A cleansing herbal combination may be used as a vaginal pack by placing it against the cervix, or as a bolus (suppository) inserted in the vagina. The pack draws out toxic wastes from the vagina, rectum or urethral areas. A "vag pac" is helpful for cysts, benign tumors, polyps and uterine growths, and cervical dysplasia. It takes 6 weeks to 6 months for complete healing to take place, depending on the problem such as the shrinking of a tumor. Co-author, Linda Page, has seen success using this method.

How to make a pack:

- Formula #1: Mix 1 part of each herb with cocoa butter to form a finger-sized suppository: squaw vine, marshmallow root, slippery elm, goldenseal root, pau d' arco, comfrey root, mullein, yellow dock root, chickweed, acidophilus powder.

- Formula #2: Mix 1 part each with cocoa butter to form a finger-sized suppository: cranesbill powder, goldenseal root, red raspberry leaf, white oak bark, echinacea root, myrrh gum powder.

Place suppositories on waxed paper in the fridge to chill and harden slightly. Smear a suppository on cotton tampon and insert, or insert as is, and use a sanitary napkin to catch drainage. Use suppositories at night; rinse out in the morning with white oak bark tea, or yellow dock root tea to rebalance vaginal pH. Repeat for 6 days. Rest for one week. Resume and repeat if necessary.

For type 2 pap smears: take green drinks daily, use CRYSTAL STAR WOMAN'S BEST FRIEND™ for 3 to 6 months; NATURE'S WAY DIM-PLUS (DIINDOLYMETHANE) 400mg daily and folic acid 800 mcg daily.

Chlamydia

The most common of all bacterial STDs, with 4 – 8 million new cases occurring each year.

After a round of antibiotics, consider CRYSTAL STAR DETOX BLOOD PURIFIER™ caps with goldenseal. Also, mix powders of goldenseal, barberry, Oregon grape root and garlic with vitamin A oil and apply directly to the inflamed cervix via an all-cotton tampon. The berberine in goldenseal, barberry, and Oregon grape helps to activate macrophage (immune eater cells) and has documented activity against chlamydia. For stubborn cases, follow up with CRYSTAL STAR ANTI-BIO™ caps with olive leaf extract or olive leaf extract caps.

Zinc 50mg 2x daily, (also mix in water and apply topically) as an immune stimulant.

STDs are a reproductive health issue that cannot be ignored.

Many men and women are opting to try safe, effective natural medicines for STDs. In my experience, natural therapies offer new hope for viral STDs, and can help produce faster recovery for bacterial and parasitic infections that require medical treatment. For healthy conception and pregnancy, appropriate STD treatment is vital for your health and that of your child.

Natural Therapies for Fibroids, Endometriosis & Ovarian Cysts

Fibroids and endometriosis are two of the biggest health complaints I hear about from women. Hardly a week that goes by that I don't get an office call or a letter from a woman who is trying to avoid fibroid surgery, or who is having problems conceiving because of a reproductive blockage. More than a half million American women have hysterectomies every year because of complications caused by fibroids and endometriosis. As many as 40% of American women 35 and older have fibroids.

A hysterectomy is the surgical removal of the uterus and sometimes the ovaries. It is major surgery, requiring a month or more of recovery time. Of course, after a hysterectomy, pregnancy is no longer an option. A hysterectomy induces a premature menopause with all of its attendant problems- hot flashes, bone loss, weight gain, and mood swings. The medical community's answer to this is usually a prescription of hormone replacement drugs that we now know are linked to breast cancer, gallbladder disease and blood clots. Most women tell me they would rather deal with the fibroids!

The majority of these problems could have been avoided. The latest research shows that only 10% of hysterectomies are medically necessary.

What are Fibroids?

Uterine fibroids are benign growths between the size of a walnut and orange that appear on or within uterine walls. Their symptoms can be mild to severe with excessive menstrual bleeding, abdominal pain, bladder infections, painful intercourse and infertility topping the list. In very rare cases, a large fibroid can block the opening to the uterus, requiring a woman to have a cesarean section if she is pregnant. Most fibroids are not cancerous, and, according to some estimates, have less than 1/2 of 1% chance of becoming cancerous before menopause. Most fibroids go away on their own after menopause. Still, for women who have them, they can be painful and cause excessive bleeding. Some fibroids make conception difficult by compressing the fallopian tubes or changing the shape of the uterus. However, many women with fibroids are able to both conceive and carry a pregnancy to term without complications.

Ovarian cysts are small, non-malignant chambered sacs filled with fluid that develop on the ovaries, usually during ovulation. They can cause pain, swelling and irregular menstruation, but generally go away on their own without any lasting effect on fertility. In some cases, cysts grow quite large and require surgery.

Polycystic Ovary Syndrome (PCOS) is another serious problem where multiple cysts develop on the ovaries and menstruation becomes irregular. Hormones, particularly testosterone, are always imbalanced with PCOS and as a result adult acne, obesity, excess facial hair and infertility commonly occur. Chronic stress and eating disorders play a role in PCOS development. The herbs, vitex and licorice, maitake mushroom, and natural progesterone cream show good results for reducing PCOS. For more on PCOS, see pg. 67. Note: Ovarian cysts have a greater likelihood of malignancy if they occur in premenstrual girls and in post menopausal women. A medical checkup is advised.

How is Endometriosis Different?

Endometriosis is caused by excess growth of endometrial tissue that is not shed during menstruation. The tissue escapes the uterus and spreads, attaching to other areas of the body- ovaries, lymph nodes, fallopian tubes, bladder, rectum, even kidneys and lungs. It grows abnormally, bleeding severely during the menstrual cycle, from the vagina or rectum, or bladder or back through the fallopian tubes, instead of normally through the vagina.

Endometriosis can mean heavy periods and pain all month long, and it increases risk for benign uterine fibroids. Endometriosis can cause major reproductive blockages, and is credited with 35-50% of infertility cases in American women.

Natural therapies can improve chances of conception by helping a woman's body normalize naturally. Simple diet changes and specific herb and supplement regimens can reduce fibroids, cysts and endometriosis.

Do You Have Warning Signs Of Fibroids, Ovarian Cysts Or Endometriosis?

A visit to your holistic physician will give you a definitive diagnosis, but two or more "yes" answers to the following symptoms should alert you to a potential problem.

- severe abdominal cramping and shooting pain; and abdominal-rectal pain
- excessive, painful menstruation; passing large clots; prolonged abnormal or irregular menstrual cycles
- chronic fluid retention, abdominal bloating
- irregular bowel movements or diarrhea during menses
- urinary frequency
- sensation of fullness or pressure in the abdomen
- ovarian swelling or severe mid-cycle pain

What Causes Endometriosis, Fibroids & Ovarian Cysts?

While scientists are still not entirely certain why endometriosis and fibroids develop, here are risk factors to be aware of:

Excess Levels of Estrogen / Deficient Progesterone: Excess estrogen fuels abnormal tissue growth and is a direct cause of fibroids, ovarian cysts and endometriosis for many women. When estrogen production declines during menopause, fibroids and other growths normally go away on their own. However, quite understandably, this isn't nearly soon enough for women who are suffering.

X-Ray Radiation: Even low dose radiation may mean increased risk for fibroids. Breast tissue is so sensitive that the time between a mammogram and fibroid growth is sometimes as little as three months.

Too Much Caffeine and Commercial Meat: Drinking 4-5 cups of coffee daily increases estrogen, triggering fibroid and cyst growth. If you like beef, you should know that Italian research reported in *Obsetrics and Gynecology* shows while eating red meat doubles the risk of developing uterine fibroids, eating plenty of vegetables cuts fibroid risk in half! Experience with the problem has me convinced that eliminating caffeine and hormone-injected meats dramatically reduces fibroid problems for many women.

Note on Oral Contraceptives: Feedback I've had from birth control users suggests that even the newest low dose oral contraceptives can cause breast and ovarian swelling, and may aggravate fibroid problems and endometriosis for susceptible women. You may want to consider alternative contraception with your physician if you're at high risk for fibroids, or if you already have them.

1. Balance Your Hormones for Fibroids, Endometriosis & Ovarian Cyst Relief

A short cleanse can really help. Start with a 24 hour vegetable juice diet to help clean out acid wastes and reduce body congestion before you try to conceive. A 24-hour detox is a juice and herbal tea cleanse that lets you go on with your normal activities, and "jump start" a healing program. Even though it's quick, without the depth of vegetable juices needed for a major or chronic problem, it's often enough, and definitely better than no cleanse at all, and can make a difference in the speed of healing.

Is your body showing signs that it needs a 24 hour cleanse?

- Do you feel "toxic"? Are you tired a lot for no reason?

- Do you feel congested? Do you have the first signs of a cold or flu? (Go right into this cleanse.)

- Is your skin dry or flaky? Is your skin tone sallow? Is your hair dull, dry and brittle?

- Are the soles of your feet or your palms often peeling?

- Do you frequently get oral herpes? yeast infections? urinary tract infections? unusual allergies?

24-Hour Detox Plan

The evening before you begin... have a green leafy salad to give your bowels a good sweep. Dry brush your skin before you go to bed to open pores for the night's cleansing eliminations. Take an herbal laxative. (not if you're already pregnant). Drink 8 to 10 glasses of water a day to hydrate, and flush wastes and toxins from all cells. Note: Avoid all liquid diets or long cleanses (more than 24 hours) if you're pregnant.

The next day: over the next 24 hours take fresh juices, herbal drinks, water, and a long walk.

On rising: take 2 tbsp. fresh lemon or lime juice, 1 tbsp. maple syrup and 1 pinch cayenne in water.

Breakfast: a fresh juice with 1 pear, 2 apples, 4 oranges, 1 grapefruit; or cranberry juice from concentrate.

Mid-morning: have a Zippy Tonic: 1 handful dandelion greens, 3 fresh pineapple rings and 3 radishes; or a cleansing, energizing green tea blend with antioxidants like Crystal Star Green Tea Cleanser™.

Lunch: juice 4 parsley sprigs, or a handful of dandelion greens, 3 tomatoes, 1/2 green bell pepper, 1/2 cucumber, 1 scallion, 1 lemon wedge; or a glass of apple juice with 1 packet chlorella granules dissolved.

Mid-afternoon: a cup of CRYSTAL STAR CLEANSING & PURIFYING TEA™ or Flora Purification tea

Dinner: take a glass of papaya-pineapple juice for enzymes; or try a High Mineral Broth: 7 carrots, 7 celery stalks, beet tops from 1 bunch, 2 potatoes, 1 onion, 4 garlic cloves, 3 zucchini, 1 handful of parsley. Place in a large soup pot, cover with water, bring to a boil, simmer 30 minutes. Remove and discard veggies.

Before Bed: have a cup of mint tea, or Red Star NUTRITIONAL YEAST Broth or miso soup.

24-Hour Detox supplement suggestions:

Cleansing boosters: CRYSTAL STAR CLEANSING & PURIFYING tea™; CRYSTAL STAR LIVER RENEW™ caps or PLANETARY BUPLEURUM LIVER CLEANSE.

Electrolyte boosters for removal of toxic body acids: ALACER ELECTROMIX; NATURE'S PATH TRACE-LYTE LIQUID MINERALS.

Probiotics: UAS DDS-PLUS, WAKUNAGA KYO-DOPHILUS; NEW CHAPTER ALL FLORA.

Vitamin C: Take 1000mg of vitamin C 3x per day with bioflavonoids.

2. After your cleanse

Follow up with a low fat, vegetarian diet. Breast swelling and painful cramping can be significantly improved within weeks after a change to a low fat, vegetarian diet.

3. Reduce caffeine

Caffeine from coffee, chocolate and colas clearly aggravate fibroids. Women with a predisposition to fibroids have a hard time metabolizing caffeine in these forms. Some women report they can consume green or white tea without any ill effect.

More on Caffeine's Link to Fibroids

- **Caffeine Increases Estrogen Levels,** a known fibroid trigger. A 2001 study reported in the journal Fertility and Sterility shows drinking just 2 cups of coffee a day boosts levels of estradiol, the natural estrogen involved in endometriosis, fibrocystic breast pain, and breast and ovarian cancer. Drinking 4–5 cups of coffee daily can wreak havoc on estrogen balance. Research shows women who consume 500 milligrams of caffeine daily, the equivalent of 4–5 cups of coffee, produce 70% more estrogen in the follicular phase of the menstrual cycle than women who consume less than 1 cup of coffee. (The follicular phase of the menstrual cycle is the period of time from the first day of menstruation until ovulation when the body strives to produce a viable follicle for ovulation.)

- **Caffeine,** especially taken at mealtimes, can also raise glucose and insulin levels, another possible fibroid trigger.

- **Coffee oils,** high in non-filtered or boiled coffee, are known to boost cholesterol levels, imbalancing body fats involved in fibroid growth.

- **From an energetic perspective,** coffee is a "heating" food that taxes the liver, disrupting hormone production and burdening the body with toxins that lead to fibroid development.

4. Rethink high-fat dairy foods like cheese, milk, and ice cream.

Naturopaths and practitioners of Traditional Chinese Medicine routinely suggest eliminating fatty dairy foods from your daily diet to reduce toxic accumulations like fibroids, fatty tumors, cysts and boils. This diet change just by itself can produce amazing fibroid relief. Cultured low-fat dairy products like yogurt and kefir, in contrast, are well tolerated in moderation.

5. Foods that are high in essential fatty acids (EFAs) are a healthy choice.

EFAs are liquid fats that help to metabolize hard, clogging saturated fats that contribute to abnormal growths. EFAs also help maintain hormone balance and reduce inflammation- important for fibroid and cyst relief. Sea greens like dulse and nori (also a good source of iodine—a proven fibroid fighter), seafoods, dark greens like spinach, cantaloupe, olive oil and avocado are healthy sources of EFAs.

6. Add cruciferous veggies like broccoli, cauliflower, cabbage and brussels sprouts.

Cruciferous veggies are one of my favorite healing foods. Indole 3 carbinole, the constituent responsible for these vegetables' unmistakably bitter flavor, is a natural antioxidant with powerful anti-tumor activity. Indole 3 carbinole improves estrogen metabolism and your body's ability to eliminate excess estrogen. New tests show that women who eat plenty of vegetables containing indole-3-carbinole may lower their risk of breast cancer. Indole 3 carbinole vegetables may also reduce fibroid and endometriosis symptoms by improving estrogen metabolism.

7. More fiber in your diet is a natural estrogen balancer.

Studies have shown that women on a high-fiber diet have lower levels of circulating estrogen. More fiber in your diet means less circulating estrogen; it reduces body congestion because excess estrogen is excreted through the bowel. Having an apple, pear or whole grain cereal every day keeps your system free flowing.

8. Watch your weight.

Maintaining a healthy weight is another key to diminish fibroids and prevent their recurrence. Fat is a storage depot for hormones and wastes that fuel fibroid and cyst growth.

Whole Herb Formulas for Fibroid, Ovarian Cyst and Endometriosis Relief

An anti-inflammatory, pain relieving formula with whole herbs can help strengthen, cleanse and normalize the ovarian-uterine area. Using this type of combination for 3 months (Discontinue if you become pregnant), especially with 2 cups of burdock tea (a liver cleanser), can help take down painful inflammation fast and help your body recover, naturally. We also recommend Evening Primrose Oil up to 4000mg daily for extra hormone balancing Essential Fatty Acids (EFAs).

CRYSTAL STAR'S WOMEN'S BEST FRIEND™ is a formula used with good results by women all over the country. It produces the best results for women with symptoms like abnormal growths with discomfort or irregular bleeding. It contains herbs such as:

Goldenseal: highly anti-inflammatory, bitter herbs that help the liver to metabolize excess estrogen

Cramp bark: specific for menstrual cramping and pain

Red raspberry: relieves cramping and normalizes the uterus; astringent activity helps normalize menstrual flow.

False unicorn: uterine and ovarian tonic that helps regulate menstruation.

For continuing natural defense, follow up with a hormone balancing formula like CRYSTAL STAR BREAST & UTERINE FIBRO DEFENSE™ for another 3 months (Discontinue if you become pregnant). This type of combination can be also helpful for symptoms of fibrocystic breasts.

BREAST & UTERINE FIBRO DEFENSE™ contains herbs such as:

Pau d'Arco: a powerful anti-tumor herb helpful for abnormal tissue reduction.

Black Cohosh: an estrogen balancer for fibroid relief. Can help normalize organ prolapses

Dandelion: helps stimulate the liver to metabolize excess estrogen. Reduces bloat, breast swelling and abdominal congestion.

Enzyme Therapy: We've talked about enzyme therapy for STDs, but protease enzyme therapy shows excellent results for fibroids and cysts. Taken between meals, it helps dissolve abnormal tissue and stimulate the immune system. CRYSTAL STAR DR. ENZYME WITH PROTEASE & BROMELAIN™ and ENZYMEDICA'S PURIFY are good choices. Dosages of 370,000 HUT or more daily are often necessary. Note: Protease may thin the blood. Ask your natural health practitioner if protease enzyme therapy is right for you.

Natural therapies can help bring your body back to health if you're suffering from fibroids, ovarian cysts and endometriosis. Your foods and lifestyle choices can be paramount in your recovery. Medical intervention may be necessary for some women with severe endometriosis and very large fibroids, but even in these cases, gentle natural therapies can guide a woman's body to faster recovery and help prevent fibroid reoccurrence.

For very large fibroids causing miscarriages, or possible complicated child labor, surgical removal (myomectomy) either by laparoscopy or by laparotomy can be a good option. If you're considering uterine artery embolization (UAE) to remove fibroids, although it can be very helpful for fibroid reduction, evidence suggests it may increase the risk of complications during a later pregnancy. Ask your physician.

When is it time to consider an infertility workup?

Infertility is defined as the inability to conceive for 12 consequent months of trying. If you are at this point, you may want to consider a workup to help understand the cause of infertility. It can allow you to target the problem and address it quicker. A workup normally includes a complete physical, sexual history, semen analysis from the man, a blood hormone evaluation for the woman, and a test showing compatibility of the man's sperm and the woman's vaginal secretions. Please note that formerly "infertile" couples have been able to conceive after following natural therapies. As we've discussed, natural therapies like acupuncture can improve your conception chances even if you're using standard methods. See pg. 40 for more. In addition, see the References section in the back of this book for couples dealing with fertility problems.

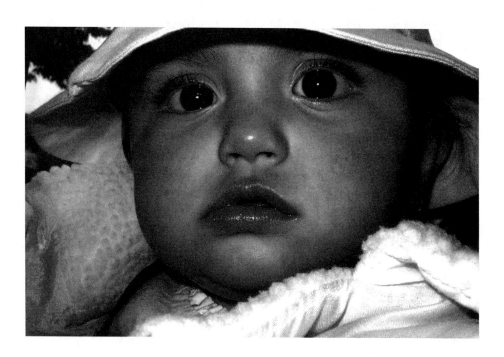

Chapter Four

Miscarriage prevention: how to improve your chances

Between 1 in 6 and 1 in 3 pregnancies end in miscarriage. Spontaneous miscarriage, most likely to occur in the first trimester, frequently happens before a woman even recognizes she's pregnant. Just 10% of miscarriages occur in women who know they're pregnant. After the first trimester, miscarriages become more rare. Miscarriage is often Nature's way of dealing with an abnormal embryo (such as development of extra fetal chromosomes, or improper fixing of the fetus to the womb walls) that could not have survived or lived a healthy life if the pregnancy had been brought to full term. There is good news though. Research suggests women who have miscarried but have had at least one child already will be able to have another successful pregnancy.

Rarely is miscarriage the fault of the mother's actions (such as stress, a fall or exercise), unless her nutrition is very poor (especially low protein, folate and trace minerals like selenium), or if she is addicted to drugs or nicotine. Even then, Nature tries hard to avoid conception under dangerous conditions. Miscarriage risk is the greatest during the first trimester, especially if the mother is over 35 and has had difficulty becoming pregnant.

Factors Involved in Miscarriage

1 in 200 women suffer from repeat miscarriages (3 or more miscarriages). In some cases, no cause can be found. However, recent research pinpoints clear risk factors that are outlined in detail here. **Work with a holistic physician to discuss your concerns and determine if you have possible risk factors.**

If a woman does not have a weak cervix, chromosomal abnormalities or autoimmune antibodies, research shows she has a 70-85% chance of carrying a pregnancy to full-term even if she's had three miscarriages.

Polycystic ovary syndrome (PCOS): Up to 10% of women who miscarry have abnormal hormone levels. (*www.salivatest.com* is an excellent resource for women who want to learn more about the status of their hormonal levels.

Imbalanced insulin levels caused by PCOS make it difficult for an embryo to attach properly to the uterus. Regulating blood sugar is a key to overcoming this problem. Too low progesterone levels don't allow for successful implantation or development. Transdermal progesterone may be as effective as progesterone injections or suppositories, and is widely available in over-the-counter supplements. PURE ESSENCE LABS FEM CREME is a good choice. Licorice and vitex extract can also normalize insulin levels for women with PCOS. The newest research shows a special extract from maitake mushroom, called Sx fraction, can reduce insulin resistance in women with PCOS, improving their chances for conception. MAITAKE PRODUCTS MAITAKE SX-FRACTION is highly recommended.

Luteal phase failure: Luteal phase failure occurs when the ovaries are unable to produce enough progesterone to allow for the successful implantation of the fertilized egg or development of the embryo. Luteal phase failure is a major cause of miscarriages, occurring in younger and younger women today, and may be the result of exposure to xenoestrogens in the womb. John Lee M.D. recommends transdermal progesterone 40mg a day to help prevent miscarriage caused by luteal phase failure. After your first month, increase dose gradually to 60mg per day. Ask your healthcare professional. Vitex extract also helps normalize ovulation for many women.

Uterine fibroids or adhesions from surgeries; abnormally shaped uterus or poor uterine muscle tone: 15% of women who have repeat miscarriages have an abnormally shaped uterus or fibroid growths that affect blood flow and successful implantation of a fertilized egg. Fibroid growths are actually more common than blue eyes, but do respond to herbal therapy in many cases. Refer to the fibroid relief program on pg. 57-65 of this book. Further, surgery may be able to correct certain types of uterine abnormalities.

Bacterial vaginosis (BV) or other chronic infection: Research from the *British Medical Journal* reveals that BV may be a cause of second-trimester miscarriages. Herbal antimicrobials like echinacea, astragalus and garlic can be helpful in these cases. Medical antibiotics, in rare cases, can lead to premature delivery.

Autoimmune antibody reaction: 11–22% of women who miscarry have a condition called **Antiphospholipid Syndrome**, which causes microscopic blood clots to develop in the blood vessels of the placenta, affecting the flow of nutrients to the baby. Early onset pregnancy preeclampsia, a history of thrombosis or heart disease, or a diagnosis of lupus or other autoimmune disease are warning signs you should be tested for Antiphospholipid Syndrome. Blood thinning medication can be helpful in these cases. Natural therapies include the use of blood thinning herbs like ginkgo biloba, white willow and turmeric, and the enzyme, nattokinase with the guidance of a holistic physician.

Embryo rejection: Embryo rejection occurs when a woman's immune system perceives the pregnancy to be a foreign pathogen which it attacks and rejects. Medical professionals now use blood tests for diagnosis, and then vaccinate the woman with the man's white blood cells before she gets pregnant.

Chromosome defects: 1 in 20 couples experience repeat miscarriage due to chromosomal defects (too much or too little genetic material delivered to the embryo). Genetic testing or in vitro fertilization can be helpful in these cases.

Cervical looseness: Relatively rare, a weak cervix that widens too early in pregnancy will likely cause miscarriage. However, this condition can be difficult to spot before pregnancy. The medical approach to this problem is suturing the cervix until the child is ready for delivery. We have personally seen a case where this technique was successful, but uncomfortable. Naturopaths suggest using herbs with tissue toning and tightening effects, like black cohosh and red raspberry during pre-conception for prevention. These are also helpful for uterine prolapse.

Diabetes: Women who have diabetes that is not controlled through diet, exercise or medication are at a greater risk for miscarriage than women with controlled diabetes. A formula like Crystal Star Sugar Control High™ can help stabilize blood sugar fluctuations, improve sense of wellbeing and strengthen the pancreas. (Use for 2 months—preconception.)

Lifestyle Factors to Avoid

Nutrient deficiency: A study in the Journal of the American Medical Association shows that pregnant women with low levels of folate, a critical B vitamin, are 50% more likely to miscarry. Folate deficiency interferes with blood flow to the embryo by increasing clotting. All women of child bearing age (and beyond) should consider a multivitamin with at least 4mg of folic acid (synthetic folate) and adding folate-rich foods like leafy green vegetables, beans, whole grains and citrus fruits to the daily diet. Preliminary research also shows selenium deficiency may be involved in some first trimester miscarriages. Women who habitually miscarry may be low in bioflavonoids.

Vitamin A toxicity: Beyond nutrient deficiency, an overload of the nutrient, vitamin A, can lead to birth defects and trigger miscarriage. Do not take more than 2500 IU of vitamin A (retinol form) in supplements. Beta carotene is a better choice, which converts to Vitamin A in the liver and is non-toxic for pregnancy needs.

Smoking: Smokers are twice as likely to miscarry and have low birth weight babies.

Drinking alcoholic beverages or a lot of caffeine: Large amounts of caffeine—4 or more cups of coffee—each day increases risk of miscarriage. Most doctors recommend their pregnant patients limit caffeine intake to 1 cup of coffee per day or 2 cups of caffeinated tea. Still, even drinking a lot of decaffeinated coffee is not a good idea. A 1996 study in Epidemiology shows drinking 3 cups of decaffeinated coffee every day was linked to increased miscarriage risk.

Non-Prescription Drugs: New research suggests that taking NSAIDs (Non-steroidal Anti-inflammatory Drugs) like ibuprofen and aspirin during pregnancy can increase miscarriage risk by 60 – 80%. In fact, physicians suggest avoiding most drugs during pregnancy to lessen negative consequences for the child.

Chemical Exposure: Toxic substances like arsenic, lead, formaldehyde, benzene and ethylene oxide can cause miscarriage. Avoid any exposure from the workplace or home. Nitrous oxide used in the dentist's office has also been linked to miscarriage. Tell your dentist if you're pregnant.

Exposure to high levels of EMFs (electromagnetic fields): Some evidence suggests that exposure to high levels of electromagnetic radiation from appliances, faulty wiring or computers can increase miscarriage risk, possibly up to 80%. The good news is that EMFs drop off quickly with distance. EMF protection suggestions:

- Avoid X-rays; they can damage the fetus.
- Use a gauss meter to determine your daily exposure to EMFs.
- Sit 2 or 3 feet away from computer monitors and hard drives.
- Stay at least 4 feet away from home appliances like TVs, microwaves, vacuums, and toasters if you're pregnant.

Stress and overwork: Women who work over 45 hours a week at stressful jobs are three times more likely to miscarry. Try to cut your hours when possible. You will become more productive and less fatigued for the hours you are working.

Avoid physical strain at the time of conception to aid implantation of the fertilized egg.

Are you at risk for miscarriage?

The first signs are spotty to profuse bleeding during pregnancy, usually with cramps, lower back pain, dizziness and severe abdominal pain. Some midwives say that if you see a lot of bright red blood, a miscarriage may not be preventable. Contact your physician or midwife right away if you're at risk. Important note: Almost 25% of women experience bleeding or spotting in early pregnancy; about half of these pregnancies continue successfully. Take a prenatal formula like PURE ESSENCE LABS MOTHER TO BE formula throughout pregnancy for a healthier baby and to help prevent miscarriage.

Natural Miscarriage Prevention

Nutritional therapy plan:

- **A good prevention/building diet should include plenty of magnesium and potassium-rich foods;** leafy greens, brown rice, green and yellow veggies, tofu, sprouts, molasses, etc. Add sea greens for natural vitamin B12 and plant protein. Be sure you get enough vegetable protein for the baby's growth: whole grains, sprouts and seeds, low fat yogurt and seafoods.

- **Avoid a restricted, raw foods diet.** Energetically, this type of diet can aggravate a "cold uterus" and stimulates downward movement. Include warming foods like nutrient-rich broths and soups, herbal pregnancy teas, whole grains, and steamed vegetables often. Skip iced drinks. Try room temperature beverages instead.

- **Limit your intake of goitrogen foods that impair thyroid function** like raw cruciferous vegetables (cooked is ok), peanuts, mustard, pine nuts, millet and soy foods, especially if you have low thyroid.

- **Avoid alcohol, caffeine, drugs.** Reduce sugars and refined foods of all kinds. NO soft drinks; they bind magnesium that reduces uterine cramping and make it unavailable.

- Mix of 1 tsp. lecithin, 4 tsp. toasted wheat germ, 1 tsp. nutritional yeast and 2 tsp. molasses; take 2 tbsp. daily over cereal or in a green drink. Note: Green drinks can be a key to a healthy pregnancy. Try ALL ONE MULTIPLE VITAMINS & MINERALS GREEN PLANT BASE daily (highly recommended) or GREEN KAMUT JUST BARLEY.

Miscarriage Preventives:

- Avoid X-rays, second hand smoke and excessive exercise.

- Use environmentally friendly household supplies whenever possible. An excess of chemicals is not good for you or your unborn child.

- When driving, place the seatbelt's lap belt below your abdomen, across your hips.

- For women at high risk for miscarriage, bed rest may be necessary.

Interceptive therapy plan:

1. Traditional help for threatened miscarriage

In every case of threatened miscarriage, contact your healthcare provider first. Lying very still and having a cup of false unicorn tea every 1/2 hour helps. As hemorrhaging decreases, give the tea every hour, then every 2 hours. Add 6 lobelia extract drops as a relaxer to the last cup. Or try a wild yam/red raspberry tea hourly; or hawthorn extract 1/2 dropperful and bee pollen 2 tsp. hourly to help control bleeding. Add natural vitamin E 500IU, every six hours to help normalize the placenta (short-term, ask your physician).

Herbal tip from talented midwife, Jeannine Parvati Baker: For threatened miscarriage due to cervical incompetence, try an herbal tea made with 1 ounce wild yam, 1 ounce squaw vine, 1 ounce false unicorn and 1 ounce cramp bark. Simmer for 20 minutes in a quart of water. Take 1 wineglass-full every four hours until symptoms cease.

In the 19th century, black haw was widely used to stop miscarriage. Today, it is still used in Europe to counteract the effects of abortion drugs.

For false labor: Magnesium therapy helps reduce false labor. If there is bleeding, go to a hospital and call your midwife. 2 capsules, cayenne, can be helpful to curtail flow. CRYSTAL STAR MUSCLE RELAXER™ caps (short term), lobelia (small amounts only) or scullcap drops can ease pain. See false labor on pg. 116-117 for more.

2. To prevent miscarriage caused by luteal phase failure or hormonal imbalance

John Lee M.D. recommends transdermal progesterone 40mg a day to help prevent miscarriage caused by luteal phase failure. After your first month, increase dose gradually to 60mg per day. Ask your healthcare professional. Progesterone therapy can also help prevent preterm deliveries. Whole wild yam creams and vitex (progesterone activity) may also help prevent miscarriage due to hormonal insufficiency. Consider PURE ESSENCE FEM CREME or Vitex extract as directed.

3. Nutritional help

Take a red raspberry, alfalfa, nettles tea combination all through pregnancy, and kelp tabs, 6 daily. Selenium deficiency may increase miscarriage risk. Make sure your prenatal includes selenium (about 60 mcg). Vitamin E 400IU can help protect against miscarriage, but discontinue a week or two before your delivery date. High doses may cause abnormal adhesion of the placenta after childbirth. Black haw tea in small doses throughout danger period helps prevent spontaneous abortion by relaxing excessive uterine contractions.

4. Vitamin C and bioflavonoids can lessen risk of pre-eclampsia and miscarriage.

Make sure your prenatal contains vitamin C (about 600mg). AMERICAN HEALTH ACEROLA PLUS with rose hips; SOLARAY QBC WITH BROMELAIN AND C are other choices (use half doses). Motherwort tea reduces anxiety.

Yoga

If you are able, try the inverted yoga postures—headstand and shoulder stand—throughout your pregnancy—especially if you're expecting twins, to help prevent miscarriage. Best done with guidance from a prenatal yoga specialist.

If you suspect miscarriage

A medical sonogram and fetal heart monitoring are recommended in every case. **If miscarriage is inevitable, seek medical or midwife guidance to ensure it is complete.** Retained tissue can cause serious infection. Abnormal vaginal discharge or a fever are infection warning signs to watch for. If blood loss is excessive, there may be signs of shock like dizziness, confusion, very pale skin or clammy skin. If shock is suspected, go to a hospital immediately.

After a miscarriage, give yourself and your partner time to recover emotionally and physically. The loss of a child brings up pain and grief for both partners. Surround yourself with people who can provide thoughtful support. Give yourself permission to grieve in your own way. It is a good idea to wait until 2–3 consecutive menstrual cycles have occurred before you try to conceive again. This also allows the uterus to regenerate and normalize at the implantation site. If you conceive again, ask your physician to test your progesterone levels to make sure they are high enough to maintain the pregnancy. Check yourself for possible risk factors, make appropriate lifestyle changes and, above all, be gentle with yourself.

Chapter Five

Pregnancy after 40 - the challenges & the rewards

If you're 40 and you want to get pregnant, you're not alone. More and more couples are making the decision to have children later in life, at a time when they are more financially secure, more prepared emotionally, and more stable within their relationship. Statistics now show that 1 in 5 women having a first child in the U.S. is over 35. In 2001, more than 450,000 babies were born to mothers between 35 – 40 years old. Women of past generations also often had children in their 40's. While pregnancy risks do increase with age, they are still quite small. Most women over 35 have normal pregnancies and give birth to healthy babies.

If you're over 35 and thinking about having children, consider these factors:

It's a good idea to get a checkup before you try to conceive. Women in their 40's are more likely to have health conditions like thryoid disorders, heart disease and diabetes which can make conception and pregnancy more difficult. Getting medical conditions diagnosed and under control can help make pregnancy more comfortable with less risks. Many pre-existing health conditions can be safely managed to reduce risk to the mother and the baby.

You may want one, but you could have two or more! Just in the last 2 decades, there has been a 59% increase in multiple births. Older moms are more likely to become pregnant with multiples. According to the *National Center for Health Statistics*, women over the age of 45 are 10 times more likely to become pregnant with multiples than women in their twenties. Our friend and colleague, Leah Thomson Viscaino was doubly blessed this year when she became pregnant with identical twin boys at age 35! Be aware that pregnancy risk factors like gestational diabetes and hypertension are slightly increased in twin pregnancies, although they can usually be managed with minimal risks to moms and babies. I personally know numerous women who have had uncomplicated twin pregnancies and deliveries.

Work with your ob-gyn to determine your personal pregnancy risk factors. Pregnancy complications like diabetes, pre-eclampsia, placental problems or developmental problems with the fetus because of smaller uterine size (intrauterine growth restriction) are increased in women over 40. In addition, older moms face a slightly higher risk for miscarriage or stillbirth, and for chromosomal defects. Proper prenatal care is critical for both older and younger moms. Stick with your prenatal vitamin regimen. Extra folic acid is the best way to prevent neural tube defects like spina bifida in your newborn no matter what your age is.

A woman at 40 also has a greater chance of having a child with Down syndrome. Yet, about 75% of babies with Down syndrome are born to women under the age of 35. Even at age 45, there's a more than a 90% chance that you won't have a child with a chromosomal disorder. Prenatal testing like amniocentesis (withdrawing a sample of the amniotic fluid) can diagnose or rule out Down syndrome, but an amniocentesis does carry risks. If you're considering prenatal testing, please see "The Pros and Cons of Amniocentesis," on pg. 78-79.

Older moms have a higher likelihood of having a Cesarean section delivery, which have longer recovery times than vaginal births. One study reports that women over 45 are 7.5 times more likely to have a Cesarean section as younger women. C-section rates are also increased with twin pregnancies, more common in older moms. However, it is important to note that the rate of Cesarean births in industrialized countries is rising partly because women are requesting them more often. In today's world, C-section delivery is not that uncommon. For more, see "What about Cesarean section (C-Section)?" on pg. 139-140.

Research shows that after age 44, a woman's fertility drops significantly. Don't wait too long if you and your partner want to have children. If you have followed the fertility enhancing suggestions in the first half of this book, and have been having unprotected intercourse on the days before and after ovulation for 6 months to one year, it is a good time to get a fertility workup. If the cause of infertility is an aging egg supply, it may be time to consider IVF with experts who can weed out eggs with abnormalities or use donor eggs. Becoming a foster parent or adopting a child are other great options that also help children in need of families. See the references section on pg. 171 for more information.

Many older moms have healthy, uneventful pregnancies. The 40's may not be the best time biologically to have a child, but there's no question that an ever growing number of people are finding that it's the best time for them socially, financially and emotionally. And, in the end, what's right for the parents is probably what's best for the child. The pregnancy diet and supplement suggestions in this book is highly recommended for older moms to stay fit and well nourished throughout their pregnancy. **For "Special Problems during Pregnancy," please see pg. 111-126.**

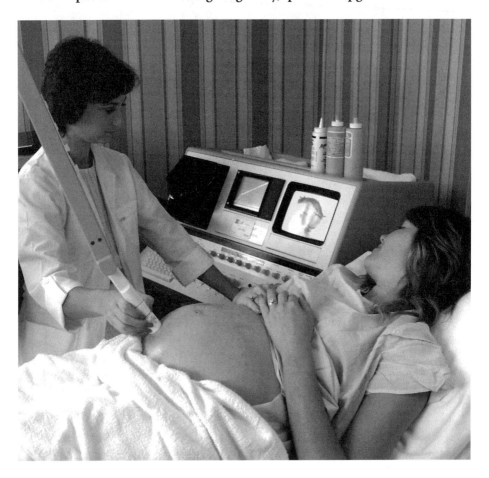

Chapter Six

Pregnancy and prenatal tests

I f you've missed one or more periods and normally have a regular cycle, there's a good chance that you're pregnant. A home pregnancy test and a visit to your ob-gyn can confirm or deny your pregnancy. Here are other body signs to watch for that you may be pregnant.

- Tender, swollen breasts
- Unexplained weight gain
- Nausea or vomiting (morning sickness)
- Fatigue
- Food aversions or cravings
- Frequent urination
- A high basal body temperature

How to take your basal body temperature

Your body temperature is a reflection of your metabolic rate, governed by the thyroid gland. Imbalances in thyroid hormone production reveal themselves in changes in basal body temperature. Normal basal body temperature is 98.6°. If your basal body temperature is chronically low, it can be a sign of low thyroid function or Wilson's syndrome. If it is chronically elevated, you could be pregnant or have a hyperactive thyroid gland (Graves disease). A visit to a physician can confirm either diagnosis.

You will need a thermometer to perform this test.

1. Before bed, shake down a thermometer to below 95°F and put it in a safe place for the night.

2. On rising, place the thermometer in your armpit for 10 minutes. Try to lie down and stay still while performing the test.

3. After 10 minutes, read your temperature and note it with the day's date.

4. Repeat your temperature test for 3-5 consecutive mornings.

Prenatal Testing

Ultrasounds use soundwaves to show a picture of your baby on a screen. Ultrasounds will be performed throughout your pregnancy to help determine your baby's age, size and once you get to 18–20 weeks, even the sex. Ultrasounds can also detect multiple pregnancies, low lying placenta and some genetic abnormalities. Your health care provider will use a hand held Doppler device to check your baby's heartbeat.

Prenatal "Triple Tests," blood tests performed during the 15–20th week of pregnancy, test hormone levels to help detect abnormalities like spina bifida or Down syndrome. If results suggest a problem, amniocentesis to confirm or rule out genetic abnormalities is usually recommended.

Testing for anemia, sexually transmitted disease, high blood pressure, HIV and urinary tract infections are also routinely performed during pregnancy to help protect the health of the mother and child.

The Pros and Cons of Amniocentesis

Amniocentesis is an elective procedure that is performed during the 15th–20th week of pregnancy to help diagnose or rule out genetic problems like Down syndrome or cystic fibrosis, and neural tube defects like spina bifida. The procedure does not detect all abnormalities, like a cleft lip or palate. Older moms whose maternal serum screening show their child is at high risk or women whose ultrasounds show abnormalities are especially encouraged to take the test. During the procedure, the physician uses a needle to pierce the amniotic sac to draw out some of the amniotic fluid. The fluid, high in fetal chromosomes, is then viewed to detect potential problems. If the amniocentesis results show there is a problem, couples can make the decision to terminate a pregnancy, if that is their choice.

In other cases, knowledge from amniocentesis testing is used to help parents be better prepared to handle a special needs child when it is time for delivery.

Amniocentesis testing is highly controversial and it does carry risks. The risk of miscarriage from this testing is about 1 in 200, unacceptably high for many hopeful parents to be. In addition, there is a slight risk of excessive bleeding, and infection or amniotic fluid leakage. In rare cases, the fetus can be injured during the procedure. Ultimately, the decision on whether to have amniocentesis is a personal one; Parents should make it with forethought and care. There is good news: About 95% of high risk women receive good news from amniocentesis results. Special note for women pregnant with multiples: Women pregnant with fraternal twins will need to have fluid drawn from each fetal sac. In the case of identical twins, one sac will need to be pierced. In either case, an amnio should only be performed by a doctor experienced with twin pregnancies.

What You Need to Know About Rh Disease

Rh disease is a disease of newborns that occurs when there is an incompatibility between the baby's blood type and the mother's. Every person has a standard blood type (like O, A, B or AB) and an Rh factor, which is either positive or negative. Rh factor is a protein that is found on red blood cells. If this protein is absent, the person is considered Rh negative, but their health is not affected negatively in any way. Around 15% of Caucasian women and 7% of African American women are Rh negative. An Rh negative woman will only become pregnant with a Rh positive baby if the father is Rh positive. Problems can occur when Rh blood types are incompatible.

During delivery, blood from the mother and baby may mix, particularly when the placenta detaches. If the mother is Rh negative and the baby is Rh positive, the mother's immune system may recognize the baby's blood as foreign and can develop antibodies against it. When this occurs, the mother is considered Rh sensitized. Rh disease does not usually occur in a first pregnancy, but may occur in subsequent pregnancies after a mother is Rh sensitized. Rh sensitization can also occur after a miscarriage or abortion.

In Rh disease, the mother's antibodies cross the placenta and attack the Rh positive red blood cells in the baby, leading to anemia, and possible jaundice and organ enlargement. At its worst, Rh disease can cause seizures, brain damage, deafness and even death in a newborn. Rh disease can be detected through amniocentesis, cordocentesis (taking a blood sample from the umbilical cord during pregnancy) and also through fetal ultrasound. Rh disease may be treated by early delivery to prevent worsening of the disease or intrauterine transfusion (through cordocentesis) of red blood cells to fight anemia. Today over 90% of treated babies with severe Rh disease survive. It is important to note that some cases of Rh disease are so mild they require no medical intervention.

How do you prevent Rh disease?

Thankfully, Rh disease is very preventable. Women with Rh negative blood are identified in early pregnancy with a simple blood test. If a women is Rh negative, she will be tested for Rh antibodies to see if she has been sensitized. If she is not sensitized, she will be given a drug called Rh immunoglobulin, which prevents sensitization in more than 95% of women. Since its development in 1968, Rh immunoglobulin has dramatically reduced RH disease in infants from 20,000 infants each year to 4,000 infants each year. If you are Rh negative, this treatment can prevent Rh disease in future pregnancies. Our friend and colleague, Leah Thomson-Vizcaino, had the Rh shot, and reported it was painless and had no adverse effects.

Gestational diabetes

Gestational diabetes, a form of glucose intolerance that occurs during pregnancy, affects nearly 100,000 women every year. It's detected through a glucose screening test that is performed after the woman is given a high sugar drink called Glucola. Some women report Glucola tastes pretty bad; others report it's not bad at all. Interestingly, research shows that eating about 18 Brach's jelly beans works just as well as Glucola for glucose screening for gestational diabetes. **Note:** New guidelines suggest women who are younger than 25, who are very thin or who are not a member of an ethnic group at high risk (Hispanic, African American, Native American, South or East Asian, or Pacific island ancestry) may not require gestational diabetes screening. Ask your physician if you're at risk and see pg.115-116 for recommendations on natural therapies to help your body rebalance.

Saving your baby's cord blood

Relatively new, and considered by some experts to be a great medical breakthrough of our time, stem cells from umbilical cord blood may be able to help your baby overcome a life-threatening disease. Banking cord blood could also help other children in your family in the event of serious illness, or even unrelated children who are sick with leukemia, immune disorders like SCIDS (bubble boy disease), or sickle cell anemia. Special stem cells in the umbilical cord can be used if your child needs a bone marrow transplant, eliminating the uncertain wait for a suitable donor. Researchers say that cord blood stem transplants may have a better safety profile than conventional bone marrow transplants.

Cord blood banking is performed immediately following the delivery of your child. It is a relatively simple procedure performed by the attending physician, nurse or technician after the placenta is delivered and after the umbilical cord is cut from your baby. It will not affect you or your child in any way during the birthing process. The cord blood is tested, processed and then stored in a cryogenic freezer for up to 21 years.

The research is still very new, but given its early successes, it may be a good idea to consider cord blood banking. Collecting and banking cord blood can cost up to $3500, but much of the expense can be paid over time. In some states, you can donate your baby's cord blood for free to help other children. In Dec. 2005, President Bush passed legislation to establish a national databank of umbilical cord blood and bone marrow to help doctors quickly find a match for patients who need a transplant. Experts are very hopeful that this vital work may some day save many lives.

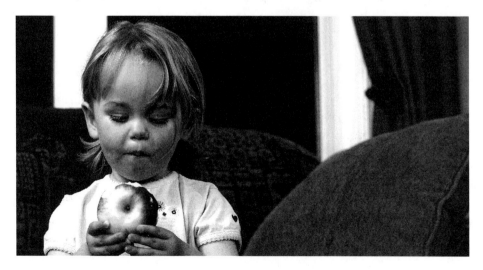

Chapter Seven

Optimal eating for two (or more)

A woman's body changes so dramatically during pregnancy and childbearing that her normal daily needs change. The body takes care of some of these requirements through cravings. During this one time of life, the body is so sensitive to its needs, that the cravings you get are usually good for you. We know that every single thing the mother does or takes in affects the child. Good nutrition for a child begins before he or she is born, actually even before conception. New research shows that when a child reaches adulthood, his or her risk for heart disease, cancer, and diabetes can be traced to poor eating habits of the parents as well as genetic factors. The nutritious diet suggestions in this section will help build a healthy baby, minimize the mother's discomfort, lessen birth complications and reduce excess fatty weight gain that can't be lost easily after birth.

A good diet also minimizes pregnancy risks and discomforts… reduces high blood pressure and fluid retention, supports your body against toxemia, helps constipation, hemorrhoids and varicose veins, gas and heartburn, morning sickness, anemia, even hormone adjustment. After pregnancy, a good diet is important for sufficient breast milk, reducing post-partum swelling, and healing stretched tissue.

Promise yourself and your baby that at least during the months of pregnancy and nursing, your diet and lifestyle will be as healthy as you can make it. A plant-based diet of whole foods along with seafood and organic poultry provide a nutritional powerhouse.

Base your pregnancy diet on whole grains, leafy greens and nutritious high protein foods. A diet with Omega 3 oils from fish, especially in the last three months of pregnancy, can increase birth weight, and lessen the risk for problems like high blood pressure later in life. New tests show high maternal levels of DHA (docohexaenoic acid, an EFA from fish) also leads to a more advanced nervous system for the infant. For example, on the first day after birth, babies with mothers who have high levels of DHA sleep more soundly than other infants, a sign of maturity and faster physical and mental development. Still, some seafoods are not safe to eat during pregnancy. Avoid shark, mackerel, tilefish and swordfish, notorious for high mercury levels dangerous to a developing fetus. See pg. 89-91 for more. A diet with turkey, eggs, legumes, nuts, seeds, vegetables, nutritional yeast (food-source B-vitamins), bananas and citrus fruits assure the best possible nutrition for your baby.

Avoid fatty animal foods like butter, beef, lamb and pork which worsen pregnancy-related symptoms like heartburn, gas and inflammation. Instead of butter, cook with small amounts of ghee (clarified butter), a nutrient rich oil with less saturated fat favored by Ayurvedic physicians during pregnancy, or olive oil. While high fat dairy foods are constipating during pregnancy, fermented dairy foods like yogurt and kefir are usually well tolerated and a good source of nutrients for the baby. (Fermented foods also guard against candida yeast infections that can be transmitted to the baby during birth.)

Avoid soft cheeses, raw milk, uncooked beef, poultry or pork, and deli meats. Wash vegetables (even organic) thoroughly before eating. Wash hands, knives and cutting boards in warm, soapy water after handling uncooked foods. Store uncooked meats away from vegetables or other ready-to-eat foods. Pregnant women are 20 times more likely to become infected with listeria (a food born bacterial illness) than other people. Listeria infection can be very dangerous during pregnancy, increasing risk for premature delivery, infection in your newborn and even stillbirth.

Avoid large amounts of soy, especially in the first trimester. High soy consumption has been linked to penis abnormalities.

Diet Keys for Prenatal Nutrition

1. **Eat small frequent meals instead of large meals.**

2. **Protein is important.** Experts recommend 60 to 80 grams of

protein daily during pregnancy, with a 10 gram increase each trimester. Most American women, even those who are vegetarian, eat this much prior to pregnancy. Focus on vegetable protein—whole grains, beans, peas, lentils, seeds, avocado, sprouts, with fish, eggs, seafood or hormone-free turkey 3 times a week. Eat high protein foods for lunch so you will be able to process them more efficiently. Take a high quality protein drink 3 times a week for optimal growth and energy. It's the quality, not the quantity of protein that prevents and reduces toxemia. Try this proven protein drink: Mix 1/2 cup vanilla rice milk, 1/2 cup yogurt, 1/2 cup orange juice, 2 tbsp. nutritional yeast, 2 tbsp. toasted wheat germ, 2 tsp. molasses, 1 tsp. vanilla, one pinch cinnamon. Two tbsp. of a high quality peanut butter from the health food store will also work just fine. **Note:** Research shows that vegetarian and vegan women have healthy pregnancies and healthy, normal sized babies. In fact, vegetarian moms actually tend to absorb nutrients more efficiently than women who eat meat.

> Did you know? A 2003 study published in the journal *Stroke* found that hunger and poor prenatal nutrition strongly correlates with stroke risk later in life.

3.   **Have a fresh fruit or green salad every day.** Eat plenty of high fiber foods, like apples, pears and prunes for regularity. Have whole grain cereals and vegetables like broccoli and brown rice for strength.

4.   **Drink plenty of healthy fluids: pure water, mineral water, and juices throughout the day to keep your system free and flowing.** Carrot juice at least twice a week is ideal. Include pineapple and apple juice. Proper hydration improves daily energy, helps prevent miscarriage, early labor, hemorrhoids, excess bleeding and dry skin.

5.   **High folate levels can help protect against birth defects** like spina bifida (incomplete closing of the spinal column that occurs in the first trimester), and first month cleft lip and palate formation. But, don't rely on fortified refined carbohydrates like commercial breads and cereals for increased folate needs during pregnancy. Eat folate rich foods: like fresh spinach, other leafy greens, sea greens, and asparagus for cell growth. Have a green leafy salad or fresh seaweed salad every day. Take 800 mcg folic acid (synthetic folate) in supplements for defense against birth defects. See pg. 92 for more information. Note: B12 is plentiful in meat, dairy products

and eggs. Vegetarian or vegan women need extra B12. RED STAR NUTRITIONAL YEAST VEGETARIAN SUPPORT FORMULA can help shore up your supply.

6.   Boost your essential fatty acids (EFAs): from fish, spinach and arugula, flax seed, and especially from sea greens (try 2 tbps. per day of dried sea greens) for your baby's healthy brain and skin. Plant oils from flax seed (BARLEANS HIGH LIGNAN FLAX OIL is our favorite), avocado, olive oil, nuts and seeds are other healthy choices. Your brain is made up of 60% fat! Avoid a diet high in saturated fats from meats and dairy; it may increase your risk of gestational diabetes.

7.   Eat carotene-rich foods: like carrots, dandelion greens or other dark, leafy greens, apricots, cantaloupe, squashes, tomatoes, yams, and broccoli for disease resistance.

8.   Eat vitamin C foods: like steamed broccoli, bell peppers and fruits for connective tissue and for allergy prevention in you and your child. Vitamin C may also be protective against certain types of childhood brain tumors linked to neural tube defects (neuroectodermal brain tumors).

9.   Eat bioflavonoid-rich foods: like citrus fruits and berries for capillary integrity.

10.   Eat alkalizing foods: like miso soup, green superfoods and brown rice to combat and neutralize toxemia.

11.   Eat mineral-rich foods, like sea veggies, leafy greens, and whole grains for baby building blocks. Include silica-rich foods for bone, cartilage, connective tissue. Many women are zinc deficient, creating potential problems for a baby's brain development. For zinc, consider foods like pumpkin and sesame seeds. Add supplemental zinc (about 15mg). Zinc may increase a baby's head circumference and weight, especially for expectant mothers who are thin. (*JAMA*, 1995) For collagen and elastin formation—try brown rice, oats, green grasses and green drinks. Blood volume goes up by 50% during pregnancy, doubling the demand for iron-rich hemoglobin. For iron, try dried fruits, green leafy vegetables, split peas, beans , blackstrap molasses or CRYSTAL STAR IRON SOURCE BLOOD BUILDER™ extract. Calcium is especially important, but should be taken at a different time than synthetic iron supplements (ferrous sulfate or gluconate). If calcium is in short supply, it will be leached from the mother's teeth and bones to help support the fetus. Eat calcium-rich green vegetables like cooked kale, broccoli or collard greens, carrot juice and carrots, and yogurt often. Calcium from herbs is a good choice, too, like CRYSTAL STAR CALCIUM-MAGNESIUM SOURCE™ and FLORADIX CALCIUM liquid.

12. **If you're craving dairy products during your pregnancy,** choose organic, low fat dairy products to avoid the antibiotic and hormone injection residues common to commercial products. Cultured dairy foods like yogurt and kefir are especially well tolerated.

13. **Include high fiber whole grains,** and fruits and vegetables to reduce excess estrogen that can affect the fetus and to stave off constipation, a common pregnancy problem. See pg.115 for more on constipation.

Sample Step-by-Step Diet for Nutritional Needs During Pregnancy

You can customize a diet like this with the vegetables, whole grains and healthy protein foods that you prefer. **Important:** Drink 8-10 glasses of pure water daily to help keep the body free flowing. Take your prenatal vitamins with meals or as directed. Have 1-2 tsp. of NEW CHAPTER GINGER WONDER syrup added to drinks daily if you suffer from morning sickness (clinically tested and good reports for nausea reduction from our testers).

On rising: Do yoga stretches and have a glass of herbal tea or room temperature water to encourage regularity.

Breakfast: have oatmeal or whole grain pancakes with yogurt and fresh fruit (sliced cantaloupe or blueberries are especially good); or poached or baked eggs on whole grain toast with a little clarified butter (ghee) and a glass of tangerine juice. If you prefer a light breakfast, try a whole grain cereal in apple or cranberry juice, the protein drink on pg. 84, or a fruit smoothie with added yogurt.

Mid-morning: have a few handfuls of organic, unsulphured dried fruit for extra iron; or have a green drink like CRYSTAL STAR ENERGY GREEN™ as a fast alkalizer (great for pregnancy toxemia and heartburn); or have a glass of carrot juice (a high calcium source) or watermelon juice (a high silica source).

Lunch: Have a chef's salad with turkey and avocado, and a baked potato with a little ghee or kefir cheese; or tuna or chicken salad sandwich with light mayo (see more on seafood on pg. 89-91) with a mixed baby greens salad with extra carrots and watercress; or a lightly seasoned red beans and rice dish with steamed or sauteed vegetables (use olive oil).

Mid-afternoon: Have an apple or pear and handful of of nuts and seeds; or have fresh, crunchy vegetables with natural peanut butter or hummus. Have a pregnancy tea: like red raspberry, nettles and yellow dock blend or EARTH MAMA ANGEL BABY HEARTBURN TEA for pregnancy-related indigestion. Or, try our friend Leah's favorite mid-afternoon pregnancy snack: NUTRABELLA BELLY BARS (highly recommended).

Dinner: Have a vegetable lasagna (use whole grain or spinach noodles) and a steamed artichoke; or have Asian stir fry with seafood, brown rice and vegetables; or have a hearty vegetable and lentil soup with steamed greens (dandelion and spinach are especially good) for extra folic acid.

Before bed: Have a cup of miso soup or a RED STAR NUTRITIONAL YEAST broth. Add a few pinches of kelp granules for extra minerals.

Important diet watchwords for pregnancy and nursing

Don't drastically restrict your diet to lose weight. Pregnancy experts in the journal *Obstetrics and Gynecology* recommend gaining between 25 and 35 pounds through the course of your pregnancy. Very thin women or women pregnant with twins may need to gain up to 40 pounds or slightly more. Women pregnant with triplets should try to gain 50 to 60 pounds! Don't skip meals. Low calories may mean low birth weight and increased risk for complications for the baby. A highly restrictive diet can affect your baby's metabolism for life!

An extra 300 calories (600 if you're having twins) daily is sufficient. You don't have to eat very much food to get those calories. Here are a few examples:

1 cup of low fat yogurt or cottage cheese = 100 calories.

1 slice of whole grain bread = 70 calories.

1 baked potato= 120 calories.

1 poached egg= 70 calories.

1 banana=116 calories.

1 mango= 132 calories.

A calorie-counting resource can be helpful. Check out: *www.calorie-count.com* and *The Concise Encyclopedia of Foods & Nutrition* By Ensminger, Ensminger, Konlande and Robson.

Limit junk foods, fats and refined foods. Avoid high sugar foods. Just the amount of sugar equal to 1 1/2 cans of soda daily increases risk for preeclampsia (pregnancy toxemia and high blood pressure) 17 times! Focus on a whole foods diet. Shop the parameters of grocery stores where the real food is, or shop in a health food store.

Eat a wide range of healthy foods to assure the baby access to all nutrients. Avoid cabbages, onions, and garlic. They can upset body balance during pregnancy. Broccoli, cauliflower, cabbage, onion, milk and chocolate (the worst!) can aggravate colic in nursing babies. Avoid red meats.

Work with a qualified health practitioner to help determine which herbs and supplements are right for you.

Don't fast—even for short periods where fasting might be helpful, like constipation, or to overcome a cold. Food energy and nutrient content may be diminished too much.

Avoid chemicalized, smoked, preserved, and artificially colored foods. Eliminate deli meats like ham, bologna and salami since they contain numerous chemicals and are a common cause of food poisoning.

Avoid caffeine (5 or more cups of coffee daily is linked to spontaneous abortion) and tobacco (linked to pregnancy complications, low birth weight, stillbirths, and SIDS- see below).

Avoid chemical solvents, and CFCs such as hair spray, and cat litter. Your system may be able to handle these things without undue damage; the baby's can't. Even during nursing, toxic amounts occur easily.

There's evidence which suggests using non-stick pans may cause birth defects or infertility. Consider stainless steel, glassware or cast iron pans for your cooking needs during pregnancy.

Avoid smoking and secondary smoke. Your baby, like you, metabolizes the harmful cancer-causing residues of tobacco. The chance of low birth weight, SIDS and miscarriage is much more likely if you smoke. Smoker's infants have a mortality rate 30% higher than a non-smoker's. Nursing babies take in small amounts of nicotine with breast milk, and become prone to chronic respiratory infections. Research shows smoking during pregnancy may also double your child's risk of having ADHD (Attention Deficit Hyperactivity Disorder).

Alcohol exposure is the most common cause of mental retardation in the U.S. More American babies are born with Fetal Alcohol Syndrome (FAS) than with Down Syndrome. Don't drink to prevent FAS, mental retardation and motor-skill problems. Even small amounts of alcohol (3 to 6 ounces daily) may increase your child's risk of Fetal Alcohol Syndrome. We recommend no alcohol at all during pregnancy.

More diet watchwords:

During labor: Refrain from solid food during active labor. Drink fresh water, or carrot juice; or suck on ice chips.

During lactation: Add almond milk, nutritional yeast, green drinks and green foods, avocados, carrot juice, goat's milk, fermented dairy like yogurt or kefir, and unsulphured molasses, to promote milk quality and richness. Fennel seed tea promotes breast milk in lactating women and reduces colic in nursing infants. EARTH MAMA ANGEL BABY MILKMAID TEA with fenugreek helps increase breast milk quickly (good results with our tester). Vitex extract also improves poor milk quality. Wayne State University studies show that exposure to pollutant PCBs from breast milk can lower a child's IQ score by as much as 6 points. Focus on organic foods to minimize exposure.

During weaning: Drink papaya juice to slow down milk flow.

Which seafoods are safe to eat during pregnancy?

Sadly, much of the seafood we have available today is high in mercury, a heavy metal released in the atmosphere naturally and by burning of industrial wastes, like fossil fuel. Mercury makes its way into our food chain from underwater volcanoes and from air pollutants in rain that are deposited in rivers and lakes. After studies showed children exposed to mercury in the womb suffered memory, attention and language problems later in life, agencies from the U.S. and the U.K. advised pregnant and nursing women not to eat large fish like tuna, shark and king mackerel, species known to contain the highest levels of mercury. Still, the most current research shows a diet high in Omega 3 fatty acids during pregnancy guards against postpartum depression, contributes to healthy eyes and brain for baby, and healthy birth weight.

I recommend wild seafood or seafood from a health food store because it is nutritious and less affected by modern food processing practices like irradiation and pesticide dumping. Yet, heavy metals like mercury in wild fish are a real concern, especially for pregnant women. Here's what you need to know about eating seafood during pregnancy.

Nearly all wild fish contain traces of mercury, but large, predatory fish contain the highest levels and present the biggest danger. High levels of mercury poison the body and can lead to nervous system damage and learning disorders in developing fetuses and young children. The newest evidence shows high levels of mercury adversely affect adults' mental performance, too. Pregnant women need to limit their mercury intake in order to protect the developing fetus. Other contaminants like DDT and PCBs which are present in some seafoods present hazards. Average about 12 ounces of cooked fish a week to limit your exposure to mercury and other contaminants.

Fish with the lowest levels of contaminants to consume safely 2 or 3 times a week are: wild salmon, shrimp, crab, butterfish, lobster (spiny/rock), freshwater trout, mahi mahi, sole, calamari, herring, scallops, halibut, and shellfish from uncontaminated waters. Eat canned fish in moderation—once a week. Canned light tuna is the lowest in mercury. Up to 6 oz. of albacore a week is ok, too.

Seafoods that are not safe to eat: Swordfish, tilefish, shark, and king mackerel present the biggest danger to pregnant women. Tuna, shark and swordfish from Connecticut are not safe for pregnant women or children either because of high mercury levels. Striped bass, rock cod, ocean perch, catfish, walleye, shark, caviar, langoustinos and Maine lobster may contain high residues of DDT, chlordane, dioxin and PCBs.

If you want to buy locally caught fish or catch your own fish, contact your local health department for advisories on the mercury level in the waters. Mercury levels vary from region to region. Stay informed about your region for more confidence when you decide what's safe for you and your family to eat.

Note 1: Avoid raw seafood unless you're positive it's parasite-free. Parasites rob you and your baby of critical nutrients needed for development. Some restaurants freeze fish before serving it raw which kills parasites.

Note 2: Farm-raised fish are more likely to contain certain contaminants (PCBs in particular) than wild fish.

To find out more about mercury contamination and mercuy in seafood, visit the National Resources Defense Council's website: http://www.nrdc. org for detailed information.

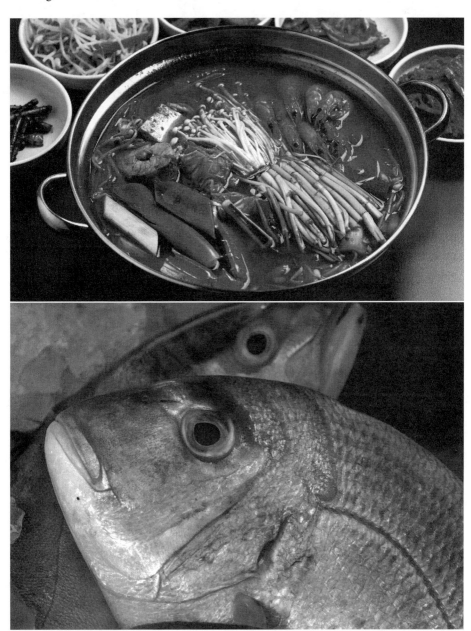

Chapter Eight

Natural pre-natal care: targeted herbs and supplements for a mother-to-be

Illness, body imbalance, even regular supplements need to be handled differently during pregnancy, even if your method is holistically oriented. A mother's body is very delicately tuned and sensitive at this time; imbalances occur easily. Mega-doses of anything are not good for the baby's system. Doses of all medication or supplements should almost universally be less (about half of normal), to allow for the infant's tiny system. Ideal supplements are food-source complexes for best absorbability.

Supplements that can help you during pregnancy

Check the label on your prenatal vitamin so you don't double up your dosages of any of the vitamins and minerals listed here. High quality prenatal vitamins will have many of the nutrients you need to supplement with during pregnancy. Work with your ob-gyn for the best results. The importance of proper prenatal care cannot be overstated.

Note: Avoid all drugs during pregnancy and nursing unless absolutely necessary. For more information, please see pg. 148-149 of this book.

…A superfood green drink. A green drink is a good nutrition "delivery system" during pregnancy because it is so quickly absorbed with so little work by the body. CRYSTAL STAR'S ENERGY GREEN RENEWAL™ drink mix or capsules contains superfoods full of absorbable, potent chlorophyllins, complex carbohydrates, minerals, proteins, and amino acids. Other good green drinks to consider: ALL ONE MULTIPLE VITAMINS & MINERALS GREEN PHYTO BASE; GREEN FOODS VEGGIE MAGMA; GREEN KAMUT JUST BARLEY.

...A good prenatal multi-vitamin supplement. Clinical tests show that mothers who take nutritional supplements during pregnancy are far less likely to have babies with neural tube and other defects. Be sure your prenatal formula contains 350 to 500mg of magnesium. Body demands for magnesium increase during pregnancy. Pre-eclampsia (marked by elevated blood pressure, fluid retention and protein loss through urine), premature labor and poor fetal growth are all tied to magnesium deficiency during pregnancy. Try PURE ESSENCE LABS MOTHER TO BE FORMULA (tested with good results), or NEW CHAPTER PERFECT PRENATAL, another healthy choice.

...Extra folic acid, 800mcg daily to prevent neural tube defects like spina bifida and anencephaly, and first month cleft lip and palate deformations. A 1999 massive nutrition study reported in *The New England Journal of Medicine* shows that supplementing with folic acid in the first 28 days of pregnancy reduces risk of neural tube defects by an astounding 85%!

Yet, even with all of the information we have, up to 33% of pregnant women do not get enough folate. Timing is essential. Supplementing folic acid after the first trimester cannot correct spinal cord damage. The March of Dimes now recommends all women of child bearing age take daily supplements with folic acid. **Fact:** Half of pregnancies that occur annually in the U.S. are unintentional!

...An absorbable, food source multi-mineral supplement with extra calcium and iron. NATURE'S PATH TRACE-MIN-LYTE , CRYSTAL STAR CALCIUM MAGNESIUM SOURCE™ CAPS, and IRON SOURCE BLOOD BUILDER™ extract all offer good body building blocks.

...Vitamin B6 50mg for nausea, vomiting, bloating, leg cramps and nerve strength; also may prevent proneness to glucose intolerance and seizures in the baby.

...Bioflavonoids daily. Low bioflavonoid levels are implicated in recurrent miscarriages. Bioflavonoids enhance vein and capillary strength, strengthen the blood vessels of the uterine wall, and help control bruising and internal bleeding from hemorrhoids and varicose veins. Bioflavonoids are a "deep tissue tonic" that support and maintain tissue integrity, tighten and tone skin elasticity. They minimize skin aging and wrinkling due to pregnancy stretching. Bioflavs are fiber-rich for regularity—a definite pregnancy advantage! Take citrus bioflavonoids 600mg with vitamin C daily, or bioflavs from herbs and gentle foods, like apricots, berries, cantaloupes, cherries, grapefruits, grapes, oranges and lemons. Bioflavonoids help control excess fatty deposits, too. Herbs and citrus fruits are some of the best bioflav sources. Bilberry extract is one of the single richest yet gentlest sources of herbal flavonoids in the botanical world, especially helpful for pregnant women suffering from distended veins, hemorrhoids, weak uterine walls and toxemia.

...**DHA,** an Omega 3 fatty acid in seafood and sea greens. Pregnant women pass large amounts of DHA in utero to their babies to ensure proper brain, eye and nervous system development. As a result, many new moms are deficient, leading to problems with forgetfulness, or even postpartum depression. In addition, DHA reserves tend to get even lower with each successive child. The DHA content of the cerebrum and cerebellum increases up to five times in the last trimester and again in the first 12 weeks after birth. We recommend HEALTH FROM THE SUN DHA liquid or NEW CHAPTER SUPERCRITICAL DHA100 to help meet high DHA demand during pregnancy. They both work! Omega 3's from flax oil is another great way to shore up EFA demands during pregnancy. BARLEANS HIGH LIGNAN FLAX OIL is a good choice.

...**Kelp tablets,** 6 daily, or CRYSTAL STAR OCEAN MINERALS™ capsules, for natural potassium and iodine. A lack of these minerals means mental retardation and poor physical development. Kelp is widely used in agriculture (animal feed) to help with fertility, healthy births and lactation, and it can help people, too!

...**Natural vitamin E,** 200-400IU, or wheat germ oil capsules, to help prevent miscarriage and reduce the baby's oxygen requirement, lessening the chances of fetal distress during labor. Note: Discontinue a week or two before your delivery date.

...**Calcium citrate with calcium ascorbate vitamin C** for collagen development. Population studies show a link between low calcium levels and pregnancy-related hypertension. Low calcium intake during pregnancy can also cause more minerals like lead to be leached from the bone which can be dangerous for both mother and child.

New research shows pregnant women who have high levels of vitamin D have babies with stronger bones. Try to get 15 minutes of early morning sunlight twice a week for healing vitamin D from sunlight.

...**Zinc,** 10-15mg daily. Statistics show half of all pregnant women are zinc deficient! Zinc deficiency results in poor brain formation, learning problems, low immunity. An Indian study reveals babies with low birth weights have significantly lower mortality rates when supplemented with zinc.

Important supplement watchwords

During the last trimester: Rub vitamin E or wheat germ oil on your stomach and around vaginal opening to make stretching easier and skin more elastic. Earth Mama Angel Baby Stretch Oil and Magia Bella Ultra-Intensive Anti-Stretch Mark Concentrate (for the belly only) are recommended. Begin to take extra minerals as labor approaches.

During labor: Take calcium-magnesium to relieve pain and aid dilation.

During nursing: Nutritional supplements like iron, calcium, B vitamins or a postnatal multiple like Pure Essence Labs Mother & Child postnatal formula, should be continued during nursing. Increase dose slightly to recover normal strength. Breast milk is a filtered food supply that prevents baby from overdosing on any one supplement. Apply vitamin E oil to ease breast crusting. Apply a marshmallow compress to relieve pressure on engorged breasts. Earth Mama Angel Baby Breastfeeding Support Kit is highly recommended to help boost milk production, fight engorgement and prevent painful, cracked nipples.

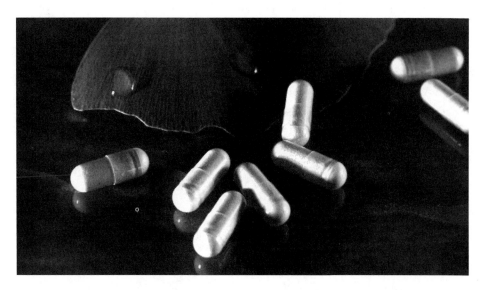

Chapter Nine

Premature labor and birth

H alf a million babies are born prematurely in the U.S. every year. Sadly, premature birth is the number 1 cause of death for newborns. One quarter of children who are born before the 32nd week of pregnancy develop problems like learning disabilities or retardation, cerebral palsy, blindness or vision impairment. Preterm babies are at risk for respiratory complications and low birth weight. Childhood asthma is more common in preterm babies. And, new evidence suggests that premature babies treated with steroids to prevent lung disease may face delayed growth and development later.

Premature labor occurs in about 11% of all pregnancies, a number that has increased by 31% since 1981! Women pregnant with multiples, who have had previous premature births or with uterine or cervical abnormalities are at a higher risk. There is some good news: Premature babies have a much better chance of survival today than ever before in history. Babies born at 32 weeks have over 95% survival rate. The survival rate for babies born at 23 weeks has grown to 40%.

The March of Dimes reports these premature labor signs to watch for:

- Contractions (your abdomen tightens like a fist) every 10 minutes or more often

- Change in vaginal discharge (leaking fluid or bleeding from your vagina)
- Pelvic pressure—the feeling that your baby is pushing down
- Low, dull backache
- Cramps that feel like your period
- Abdominal cramps with or without diarrhea
- A feeling of unease and great fatigue

Watchwords to guard against preterm labor

Drink plenty of fluids. Dehydration increases risk of premature contractions.

Take your multivitamins. Research from the *American Journal of Epidemiology* shows women who take multivitamins before becoming pregnant are less likely to give birth prematurely. DIAMOND FORMULAS HEALTHY HORIZONS is a good choice before conceiving. After conception, try PURE ESSENCE LABS MOTHER TO BE formula or NEW CHAPTER'S PERFECT PRENATAL.

Consider a DHA supplement. Low DHA levels can increase risk for preterm and low birth weight babies. I like HEALTH FROM THE SUN'S ULTRA POTENT DHA LIQUID. Eating DHA-enriched eggs can also decrease the incidence of preterm and low birth weigh babies.

Lifestyle factors to avoid: Alcohol, drugs, nicotine and second hand smoke. Poor nutrition, high stress, domestic violence, long working hours (especially long hours standing), all increase risk of preterm labor. Problems with the placenta, infections, and genetic and metabolic disorders increase preterm labor risk, too.

If you think you're experiencing premature labor, call your healthcare provider and go to a hospital. Monitor your contractions so you can report them to your ob/gyn. Emptying your bladder, drinking a few glasses of water, and lying down on your left side can be helpful. Avoid lying flat on your back; it can increase contractions. Your doctor will be able to tell if your cervix is dilated, a clear sign of premature labor. However, premature labor does not always result in delivery. Many times, the contractions can be stopped and bed rest can help a mother carry to term. About a quarter of all preterm births are intentional, but labor will only be induced early if a woman develops very severe preeclampsia, other illness or if the baby stops growing.

A special note to Moms on bed rest

Women who have signs of early labor or who are pregnant with multiples may be advised to go on bed rest. Bed rest takes advantage of the healing power of gravity. Lying down reduces pressure on the cervix, which helps prevent uterine contractions and preterm labor. By limiting physical exertion, bed rest limits stress on the heart, kidneys and circulatory system. Lying down also improves blood flow to the uterus, so the babies will receive even more nutrients from your food. Many moms-to-be dread the thought of so much idle time in bed, but you can use bed rest to your advantage by exploring new hobbies that challenge your mind instead of your body.

Get creative: While we admit we love Netflix, we don't recommend watching TV or movies 24/7 during bed rest. Bed rest is a great time to explore your inner artist. Try craft projects like scrapbooking (setting up scrapbook photo album pages for baby's arrival is one idea). Knitting, coloring, and artwork are other fun craft projects to try.

Read: Experienced moms remind us that after the baby is born you'll have less time for reading. It's a great time to finish that novel you've been putting off. Leah recommends perusing Mothering and Parenting magazines for tips that you can really use after the baby is born. Reading our special section "After Your Baby Is Born" is another good idea.

Get connected: Use a laptop to connect with other pregnant women on bed rest. *Babycenter.com, Parentsplace.com* and *Yahoo.com* all have online groups you can join to share your pregnancy experiences.

Be patient and stay centered: Spiritual practices like prayer, meditation and guided imagery help ease fears and help you visualize a healthy delivery.

Focus on your health: drink plenty of fluids, eat foods recommended in the pregnancy diet section and remember to take your pregnancy supplements and prenatal vitamins.

Sex during pregnancy

Having sex during a normal pregnancy is very safe. Some women's libidos go into overdrive during pregnancy. Increased blood flow and enhanced skin sensitivity recharges the sexual experience for many women.

But before you get excited, not all pregnant women experience this libido surge. Some women may feel uncomfortable, fatigued or simply not in the mood for sex while pregnant. One or both partners may be uncomfortable with the idea of sex during pregnancy. Some couples are concerned that sexual activity will hurt or affect the child adversely.

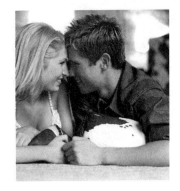

In a normal pregnancy, your baby is well protected in the amniotic sac and by your uterine muscles. Further, a thick mucous plug which seals the cervix guards against possible infection from a man's sperm. Having sex can be healthy for the majority of pregnant women. Having an orgasm is a natural Kegel! Orgasms actually strengthen the vaginal muscles and help prepare your body for childbirth, without leading to premature labor or birth.

If you're in the mood, you may need to experiment a little to see what is most comfortable. Having sex in the "spooning" position is one suggestion. Don't worry if your baby becomes more active right after sex; your increased heart rate can cause a temporary increase in activity for the baby.

Here are situations when it is not a good idea to have sex during pregnancy:

Avoid sex during pregnancy if you:

- have a high-risk pregnancy
- have a history of miscarriage or preterm birth
- your water has broken
- you have a weak or dilated cervix
- you have unusual symptoms like cramping or vaginal discharge
- you have an STD outbreak like herpes lesions or genital warts
- have placental abnormality like placenta previa. (In placenta previa, the placenta lies low, covering the cervix partially or completely. Having intercourse with this condition could cause to heavy bleeding and preterm delivery. In placenta previa, a cesarean delivery is usually necessary.)

Chapter Ten

Herbs for a healthy pregnancy

Good and easy for you; gentle for the baby.

Whole herbs can be used to ease the discomforts of hormone fluctuations, stretching, bloating, and nausea without impairing the baby's health. Clinical research shows herbs like red raspberry, ginger and echinacea are safe when used properly during pregnancy. Many other herbs have been used traditionally by midwives and naturopaths with excellent results for centuries, but small herb companies simply lack the funding for double-blind studies to scientifically demonstrate their results.

A study in *Obstetrics and Gynecology* 2001 reports that 91% of the women surveyed were using herbal remedies during pregnancy. Around one-fifth of pregnant women take some form of raspberry leaf! Whole herbs are mineral-rich foods, perfect for the extra growth requirements of pregnancy and childbirth. They are easily-absorbed and non-constipating. Ideal supplements for a developing child's body should be from food source complexes. Herbs are identified and accepted by the body's enzyme activity as whole food nutrients, lessening the risk of toxemia or overdose, yet providing gentle nutrition for both mother and baby.

The best pregnancy herbs offer very gentle healing activity. They can be used as culinary herbs added to recipes and taken as teas, both very safe delivery systems. I've provided a detailed list of healthy pregnancy herbs with suggestions on the following pages. Herbs with powerful cleansing, laxative, blood moving (emmenagogue) or abortifacient activity should be avoided. See a detailed list of the herbs that are contraindicated during pregnancy on pg. 106-107.

Important: If there is any question, always use the gentlest herbs and consult your ob-gyn or midwife. See our notes on early pregnancy and late pregnancy, which are considered separately with medicinal herbs.

Herbs you can take during pregnancy

Many women prefer body balancing teas during pregnancy. They are the gentlest way to overcome morning sickness and hormone adjustment. Take two daily cups of red raspberry tea (high in iron, calcium and other minerals); EARTH MAMA ANGEL BABY MORNING WELLNESS TEA (for nausea) or EARTH MAMA ANGEL BABY THIRD TRIMESTER TEA (only for third trimester) to strengthen the uterus and birth canal, guard against birth defects, long labor and afterbirth pain, and tone the uterus for a quicker recovery.

Iodine-rich foods are a primary deterrent to spinal birth defects. Consider kelp tablets, a sea greens sprinkle, CRYSTAL STAR OCEAN MINERALS CAPS™, or NEW CHAPTER OCEAN HERBS.

Many pregnant women need extra calcium and iron, minerals that are easily depleted during pregnancy. Herbal sources of calcium and iron are one of the best ways to get these minerals because they absorb through the body's own enzyme system. Herbal minerals provide the best bonding agent between your body and the nutrients it is taking in. They are also rich in other nutrients that encourage the best uptake by the body. Consider CRYSTAL STAR CALCIUM MAGNESIUM SOURCE™, a calcium-magnesium rich compound of whole herbs for optimum uptake, and naturally-occurring silica from herbs like oatstraw, nettles and dark greens to help form healthy tissue and bone—a prime factor in collagen formation for connective and interstitial tissue. CRYSTAL STAR IRON SOURCE BLOOD BUILDER™ EXTRACT drops in warm water, or FLORADIX IRON PLUS HERBS are absorbable, non-constipating herbal iron sources with measurable amounts of calcium and magnesium, along with naturally-occurring vitamins C and E for optimum iron uptake.

Consider a mineral-rich pre-natal herbal compound during the 1st and 2nd trimester, for absorbable minerals and toners to elasticize tissue and shore up nutrients. A good formula might include herbs like red raspberry, nettles, oatstraw, alfalfa, chamomile, peppermint, yellow dock root, and dairy free acidophilus (Try UAS DDS PLUS or JARROW JARRO-DOPHILUS). During the last trimester, we recommend a broad activity herbal mineral compound, like CRYSTAL STAR OCEAN MINERALS™ CAPS, or CALCIUM-MAGNESIUM™ CAPS, loaded with highly absorbable plant minerals, or FLORADIX CALCIUM-MAGNESIUM liquid with vitamin D, zinc and herbs.

Five weeks before the expected due date, an herbal formula to help your body prepare for labor, aid in hemorrhage control and uterine muscle strength for correct presentation of the fetus might contain herbs like red raspberry, false unicorn, cramp bark, squaw vine and bilberry. A simple raspberry leaf tea used in the last trimester helps soften the cervix in preparation for childbirth and stimulates milk production. EARTH MAMA ANGEL BABY THIRD TRIMESTER TEA is good choice for mineral nutrition from herbs and uterine tone.

Herbs you can take during labor

EARTH MAMA ANGEL BABY LABOR EASE TEA, RED EARTH HERBAL DROPS LABOR-EASE DROPS (birthing formula- use with midwife guidance), or CRYSTAL STAR PMS RELIEF™ DROPS for fast acting relief of contraction pain. Put 15 to 20 drops in water and take small sips as needed during labor. Try CRYSTAL STAR STRESS OUT MUSCLE RELAXER™ drops in warm water for afterbirth pain (excellent results), an analgesic formula that helps the lower back and spinal block area, often within 20 minutes.

Experienced moms tell us over and over again that light yoga or pilates exercises, and breathing exercises (lamaze) are invaluable for labor preparation. Don't forget to schedule your childbirth education classes a few months before the birth.

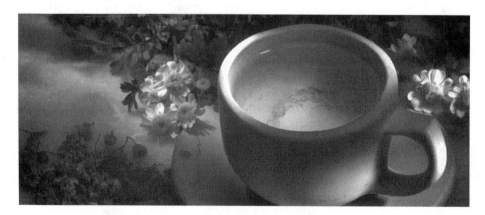

Herbs for a healthy pregnancy

Unless otherwise specified in this section, consider taking these herbs in the mildest way, as relaxing teas, or as directed by your clinical herbalist, midwife or other health care professional during pregnancy. Always discuss the herbal remedies you are taking with your ob-gyn or midwife.

Alfalfa: highly nutritive, rich in enzymes, full of vitamin K to support proper blood clotting and reduce postpartum hemorrhage. A good vegetarian source of protein and iron. High in vitamins A, D, E and B6, trace minerals, and calcium and magnesium. High in chlorophyll with gentle cleansing properties.

Bilberry: a gentle astringent herb, rich in bioflavonoids to fortify veins and capillaries. A hematonic for kidney function and a mild diuretic for bloating. Just 10-15 drops of the extract diluted in hot water works well.

Black and blue cohosh: used to assist child labor and delivery, and in the final weeks of pregnancy for labor preparation. Blue cohosh also has a reputation for normalizing contractions for false labor. To avoid risks, use both herbs only with guidance from a clinical herbalist, experienced midwife or naturopath.

Black haw: interchangeable with cramp bark, relaxes uterine muscles for women at high risk for miscarriage, relieves pregnancy leg cramps.

Burdock: mineral-rich, hormone balancer, liver booster. Reduces water retention and may prevent baby jaundice. Helpful for pregnancy-related urinary tract infections. A mild blood/liver purifier for infections like herpes. Also reduces itchy skin from belly expansion.

Chamomile: relaxes for quality sleep, lifts the spirit, improves morning sickness, and helps digestive and bowel problems. A nervine tonic high in potassium and calcium. Reduces gas and indigestion. Not for women allergic to ragweed.

Cramp bark: interchangeable with black haw, relaxes uterine muscles for women at high risk for miscarriage, relieves pregnancy leg cramps.

Dandelion leaf (fresh or dried) and root: a gentle diuretic that reduces pregnancy-related water retention; reduces fatigue, system sluggishness and constipation. A high source of vitamin A, calcium, potassium and iron. The root is especially good as a gentle liver tonic. Dandelion greens are another choice that provide premier nutrition.

Dong quai root: a blood nourisher, rather than a hormone stimulant. Use in moderation.

Echinacea: an immune system stimulant to help fight colds, flu and infections. A 2000 study by Gallo et. al. showed echinacea use during pregnancy was not associated with an increase in birth defects.

Evening Primrose oil: provides high quality vegetarian EFAs and can help soften the cervix in preparation for labor in late pregnancy.

False unicorn: used for miscarriage prevention with cramp bark, wild yam and squaw vine. Use with guidance from a clinical herbalist, experienced midwife or naturopath.

Ginger root: excellent for morning sickness, gas and indigestion; has lots of needed minerals and carminative properties (gas relieving). Ginger works best in its whole form for morning sickness. A 1991 scientific review found no reports of birth defects or miscarriage from ginger. Use by itself in a tea or with spearmint, orange peel and chamomile. In one study of women with severe morning sickness (hyperemesis gravidum), just 250 mg. of ginger taken four times a day reduced nausea and vomiting for 70% of subjects tested. Note: The FDA states that taking up to 5 grams of ginger is safe as a food. Just one gram is sufficient as a morning sickness remedy.

Lady's mantle: a uterine tonic with astringent properties for diarrhea. Can help reduce risk of hemorrhaging during childbirth. Use with guidance from a clinical herbalist, experienced midwife or naturopath.

Lavender: a relaxing, anti-stress nervine for anxiety and insomnia. Helps reduce mild depression and panic attacks. Add 1/4 tsp. lavender to your favorite pregnancy tea or include a cloth bag of the blossoms in a warm bath before bed. Lavender pillows also work nicely.

Lemon Balm: high in vitamin C for collagen development. Helps relieve irritability and mild depression. Gentle anti-allergy activity. Increases energy, improves mood and normalizes digestive health.

Marshmallow root: very mucilagenous to soothe mucous membranes. A specific for pregnancy-related heartburn, especially in combination with chamomile and slippery elm. Also helpful for bronchitis or coughing during pregnancy.

Nettles: a very mineral-rich herb, with vitamin K to guard against excessive bleeding and iron to guard against anemia. Supports healthy kidney filtration and helps prevent hemorrhoids. Enriches milk quality. High calcium in nettles helps diminish leg cramps and childbirth pain, too.

Nutmeg, sage, and parsley: safe to use in small amounts in cooking. Note: Avoid large doses of these herbs. Nutmeg can be toxic at high levels. Sage and parsley have emmenagogue activity in high amounts.

Oats & Oatstraw: sources of calcium and magnesium to prevent leg cramps, reduce anxiety and aid baby's development.

Peppermint, Spearmint: helps digestion, soothes the stomach and overcomes nausea and gas. Contains highly absorbable amounts of vitamin A, C, silica, potassium and iron. Just a few cups of tea works well. Avoid very strong preparations or high doses.

Red Raspberry: the quintessential herb for pregnancy. Rich in needed nutrients like calcium, iron, potassium, and vitamins B, C and E. An all around uterine tonic. It is anti-abortive to help prevent miscarriage, antiseptic for protection against infection, astringent to tighten tissue, rich in calcium, magnesium and iron to help prevent cramps and anemia. It facilitates birth by improving natural contractions, and is hemostatic to reduce risk of hemorrhaging. Note: Red raspberry does not increase risk of preterm contractions or labor. Some women report that taking red raspberry throughout pregnancy significantly reduces labor pain during childbirth. Assists with plentiful milk production, too. Preliminary research from the U.K. reveals red raspberry is an effective pregnancy tonic for women. Try red raspberry by itself or in combination with other herbs like spearmint, nettles and ginger as a gentle tea three times a day. EARTH MAMA ANGEL BABY MORNING WELLNESS TEA is a good choice.

Rose hips: rich in vitamin C for collagen production.

Sea greens like kelp, dulse, sea palm and nori: exceptional source of vitamins and minerals to prevent birth defects; balances thyroid.

Slippery Elm: eases constipation, soothes mucous membranes of GI tract. Helpful for morning sickness, especially taken as a hot cereal when other foods aren't well tolerated. Use inner bark only.

Squaw vine: a valuable herb for late pregnancy. Use in combination with red raspberry, nettles, spearmint and oatstraw in a tea during the last trimester to help the uterus prepare for labor. I recommend EARTH MAMA ANGEL BABY THIRD TRIMESTER TEA.

Wild yam: for general pregnancy pain, nausea or cramping; lessens chance of miscarriage.

Yellow dock root: in small amounts, it improves iron assimilation and helps prevent infant jaundice. In large amounts, it has laxative activity and should be avoided.

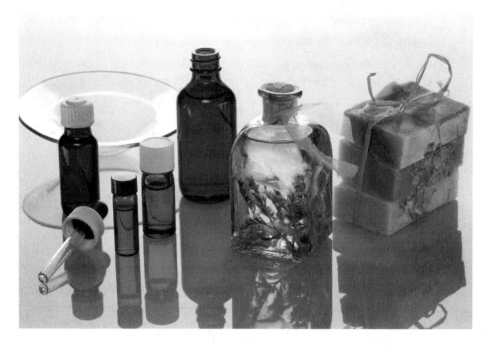

Aromatherapy

Essential oils of lavender and chamomile alleviate nausea (dilute first, and use in an aromatherapy diffuser). Lavender oil also works well diluted with a carrier oil like grapeseed oil used topically to heal perineal tears after childbirth. I recommend EARTH MAMA ANGEL BABY NEW MAMA BOTTOM SPRAY. Do not use essential oils internally during pregnancy.

Aromatherapy essential oils of fennel seed and anise reduce heartburn (dilute first and use in an aromatherapy diffuser).

Herbs to avoid during pregnancy

Medicinal herbs should always be used with common sense and care, especially during pregnancy. Some herbs are not appropriate. The following list highlights some of the herbs that are known to be contraindicated or cautioned against during pregnancy. If you're unsure or are considering using an herbal formula or single herb which is not discussed in this book, consult with a clinical herbalist or other healthcare professional first.

Contraindicated, cautionary herbs

Aloe vera: can be too strong as a laxative. Dilute aloe vera juice with 4 parts water if you decide to use it, or use an aloin-free brand like Herbal Answers Herbal Aloe Force juice.

Angelica and rue: stimulate oxytocin that causes uterine contractions.

Barberry, butternut, buckthorn, cascara sagrada, mandrake, rhubarb root and senna: too strong as laxatives.

Black cohosh, blue cohosh: can stimulate uterine contractions. Blue cohosh also affects uterine sloughing. (Both herbs are used to help child labor progress, but they should be only used with guidance from a clinical herbalist, experienced midwife or naturopath. See previous.)

Buchu, juniper and uva ursi: too strong diuretics.

Coffee: too strong a caffeine and heated hydrocarbon source—an uterine irritant. In extremely sensitive individuals who take in excessive amounts, it may cause miscarriage or premature birth.

Coltsfoot: may poison the fetus.

Comfrey: pyrrolizides (carcinogenic) cannot be commercially controlled for an absolutely safe source. Topical preparations are safe and beneficial.

Ephedra, Ma Huang: contains ephedrine alkaloids that can overstimulate the heart and cardiovascular system.

Goldenseal, lovage, mugwort, southernwood, wormwood: emmenagogues that cause uterine contractions. **Mistletoe, birthwort, cotton root, thuja, tansy and wild ginger** also act to cause uterine contractions.

Horseradish: too strong for a baby.

Hyssop: its volatile oil is too strong for a developing fetus.

Licorice root: can exacerbate water retention and high blood pressure in susceptible persons. In large amounts, licorice may lead to preterm deliveries.

Male fern: too strong a vermifuge.

Pennyroyal: stimulates oxytocin that can cause abortion.

Scotchbroom: can overstimulate the heart and cardiovascular system.

Yarrow and shepherd's purse: strong astringents and mild abortifacients.

Herbs you can take during nursing

As a general rule, the same herbs that are safe to use during pregnancy are safe while nursing. This helps ensure that the baby is only exposed to the most nutritive and gentle of all herbs both in utero and postpartum. You can also use specific herbs (galactagogues) to enrich milk quality or help in the weaning process, but some of these herbs should only be used postpartum. See the following list for notations on pregnancy contraindications. Use herbs for nursing as gentle teas unless otherwise specified. Here are a few of the best remedies we've worked with:

Alfalfa: mildly estrogenic herb that enhances milk production. Add alfalfa sprouts to salads and include a green drink daily with alfalfa like **All One Multiple Vitamins & Minerals** green phytobase daily. Safe to use during pregnancy.

Blessed thistle: a bitters herb that supports the liver and boosts milk production. Best used as a tincture. 10–20 drops, 2–3 times daily is a good daily dosage. Add to hot water to reduce alcohol content. Not for use during pregnancy as it has emmenagogue properties (stimulates menstruation).

Fennel seed: Adding fennel seed to a lactation tea can increase milk production and reduce colic, indigestion and flatulence in your baby. Fennel seed is also useful for colds in babies because it helps dissolve mucous in the upper respiratory tract. Use the seed, not the oil. Safe to use in moderation during pregnancy (tea combinations are best) and especially helpful for indigestion and gas.

Fenugreek: helps keep baby colic free while promoting breast milk flow. Note: fenugreek use can cause a new mom to smell like maple syrup, but this is a temporary reaction and should not be a cause for concern. Use fenugreek in herbal tea combinations like Earth Mama Angel Baby Milk Maid tea or Motherlove More Milk Plus extract (both tested highly effective). Not for use during pregnancy in amounts other than those used in cooking. At higher dosages, fenugreek can stimulate uterine contractions.

Goat's rue: helps to build mammary tissue, particularly helpful for women with PCOS (Polycystic Ovarian Syndrome), adoptive mothers or women who have had breast reduction surgery who want to breastfeed. Not for use during pregnancy.

Hops: great for new moms of multiples who need more milk. Try a cup of hops tea before bed to ease sleep and increase milk production for frequent nighttime feedings. Add a little brown sugar, cinnamon, ginger, mint or orange peel to taste. Drinking one alcohol-free beer rich in hops daily is another good choice. Hops is best used postpartum rather than during pregnancy due to estrogen-like effects.

Marshmallow: a mucilaginous, nutritive herb that makes breast milk sweeter and richer for the baby. Some mothers report that marshmallow helps their babies feel more satisfied after feedings. Safe throughout pregnancy.

Nettles: good source of plant iron for restoring strength after pregnancy, nettles also increases milk production and flow. Safe throughout pregnancy.

Red raspberry: used after birth, it can help decrease uterine swelling for faster recovery, and increase milk production. Because it gently cleanses and purifies the blood, it provides helpful detoxification for new moms without putting undue stress on the baby. Safe throughout pregnancy.

Vitex extract: can help promote an abundant supply of mother's milk. In one study, vitex significantly improved milk flow and milk-release for nursing women when compared to placebo. Best used if milk flow is low after childbirth.

More nursing tips for new moms

Eat carotene rich foods every day to boost lactation: sweet potatoes, carrots, green beans, asparagus, kale, collard greens, apricots, dandelion greens, watercress and asparagus. Have a handful of roasted sesame seeds for extra calcium and vitamin E. Add 2 tbsp. nutritional yeast to your daily diet for extra B vitamins to promote and enrich milk.

Just 1 – 2 tbsp. of iodine-rich sea vegetables daily helps promote mineral rich breast milk.

Take HEALTH FROM THE SUN ULTRA POTENT DHA to enrich breast milk with critical brain boosting EFAs for baby's development.

For infants with mild jaundice, HYLAND'S NATRUM SULPHURICUM tabs as a safe and natural homeopathic liver remedy. Breastfeeding a few times a day near a well lit window will help overcome mild infant jaundice. More severe cases may require phototherapy treatment. Ask your physician.

Adding a little chamomile and lemon balm to your nursing teas will also help calm and soothe a fussy baby without great risks or side effects.

Immune boosting antibodies in breast milk are dramatically reduced after vigorous workouts. Feed your baby before and one hour after workouts for the best results.

Herbs you can take for weaning

A parsley-sage tea can help dry up milk. MOTHERLOVE SAGE EXTRACT is another good choice. Dosage: Take 3 – 4 drops per ten pounds of nursing mother's body weight every three hours to decrease milk supply. Not for use during pregnancy.

AMAZAKE rice drink can help wean baby from breast milk. Use with a conventional formula for the best results. AMAZAKE is not a substitute for breast milk, but it is very nutritious and nourishing for older babies who are being weaned.

Can I color my hair during pregnancy?

Experts suggest avoiding chemical hair treatments like perms or relaxing treatments during pregnancy to protect your baby from chemical exposure. But what about hair color? Experts once recommended avoiding all color treatments during pregnancy. But, newer products have a better safety profile, and some can be used during pregnancy with knowledge and care. Ask your stylist about the safest products that are available today for pregnant women. Ask your physician about hair treatments during pregnancy, too.

If you decide to color your hair, I recommend doing it after your first trimester in a well vented room and using products with the most natural ingredients. Vegetable-based products, such as henna, are very safe, and add a reddish hue some people love. HERBAVITA'S HERBATINTS are another good choice; TINTS OF NATURE brand uses natural organic ingredients with no harsh ammonia. Read labels carefully, and avoid products with high retinols and bleaches.

Good to know... Hormonal changes during pregnancy may mean your hair color could turn out differently than usual.

Chapter Eleven

Special problems during pregnancy

P regnancy is a very personal, unique experience. Every woman will have her own set of symptoms... a big reason why there are so many old wive's tales passed from generation to generation. Some pregnant women will have beautiful, clear complexions; others may experience more acne or pigmentation problems. (Our friend and colleague, Leah, reports that for her, "The pregnancy glow is a lie!") Half of pregnant women have morning sickness in the first trimester; others feel simply fatigued or moody. Pregnancy also brings digestive issues for many women: gas, heartburn and constipation plague pregnant women in droves. Still, some women with chronic diarrhea from I.B.S. (Irritable Bowel Syndrome) actually experience relief during pregnancy because of dramatically increased progesterone levels.

Almost universally, the last month of pregnancy is challenging, with regular discomfort from a near full term baby competing for space with your internal organs (ouch!), difficult sleep, and itchy skin from belly expansion. Further, while many women have uncomplicated childbirths, others may require medical treatments to help. Wherever you fall in this scale, you can use the recommendations in this book as a helpful tool on your journey to motherhood.

Here are the main complaints we've heard from the pregnant women we've worked with, and the best ways to prevent or reduce them with gentle natural therapies that are healthy for you and your baby.

Note: Always consult with a physician or experienced midwife before using natural therapies during pregnancy.

Afterbirth Pain

Childbirth is taxing to the muscles of a woman's pelvic floor. Pain and soreness can occur for a few weeks to a month after delivery. If you get an episiotomy, you'll probably need even longer to heal the vaginal stinging and discomfort.

Take CRYSTAL STAR STRESS OUT!™ extract and CALCIUM MAGNESIUM™ caps, especially after a long labor, to relax uterine contractions and pain; EARTH MAMA ANGEL BABY POSTPARTUM RECOVERY tea to restore vitality, tone the uterus and reduce tension; una da gato tea for quicker return to normal. Take bromelain, 1500mg to relieve swelling. For post-partum tears and sore perineal muscles, use a sitz bath: 1 part uva ursi, 1 part yerba mansa root, and 1 part each comfrey leaf and root. Simmer 15 minutes, strain, add 1 tsp. salt, pour into a large shallow container; cool slightly. Or use MOTHERLOVE'S SITZ BATH or EARTH MAMA ANGEL BABY POSTPARTUM BATH HERBS. Sit in the bath for 15 to 20 minutes twice daily. Use EARTH MAMA ANGEL BABY NEW MAMA BOTTOM SPRAY to aid healing from episiotomies and perineal tears.

Anemia

Iron needs double during pregnancy due to increased blood volume.

Take a non-constipating herbal iron, like PURE PLANET SPIRULINA, diluted yellow dock tea, CRYSTAL STAR IRON SOURCE BLOOD BUILDER™ extract in hot water, or FLORADIX IRON plus herbs. Have a green drink often, such as apple-alfalfa sprout-cucumber juice, GREEN FOODS CARROT ESSENCE. Add vitamin C and E to your diet, eat plenty of dark leafy greens.

Backache

During pregnancy, the weight of the baby and stretching of ligaments often cause back pain, especially during the last trimester.

Try St. John's wort extract every few hours as needed (short term). Add 5-10 drops of Scullcap for maximum benefits. Apply BAYWOOD TOPICAL SUPER COOL RELIEF for pain reduction (highly effective). Prenatal yoga exercises help to alleviate pressure and discomfort. Watch posture and wear flat, comfortable shoes. Before bed, elevate your feet on pillows to fight ankle swelling and reduce pressure on your back.

Bladder Infection/Yeast Infection

UTI's and yeast infections can go hand in hand during pregnancy. Higher glucose levels in urine can trigger bacterial overgrowth. In addition, more urine collects in the urinary system, leaving women more susceptible. Yeast infections are also more common in pregnancy than any other time in a woman's life, especially in the second trimester.

Avoid powerful anti-fungals and antibiotics; they are too harsh for the baby's tiny system. Try simple home remedies instead. For UTI's: the simple sugar, D-mannose flushes out bacteria for fast relief, 1 teaspoon every 2-3 hours until symptoms clear (ok for diabetics, too). Drink a lot of water, 48 to 64 ounces daily, and have cranberry juice with no added sugar. For candida yeast overgrowth: Avoid sweets, fruits and fruit sugars, and yeasted breads until infection clears. Have organic yogurt daily and apply plain yogurt topically to the external vaginal area for relief. Supplemental probiotics fight candida. Finnish research shows probiotics also enhance immune response during pregnancy and may even prevent childhood eczema in your baby. I like UAS DDS-Plus.

Breasts

Breast pain, engorgement and incredible tenderness are common problems for nursing moms. Breastfeeding can be hard work, but it is well worth it. For mom, nursing helps cement her bond with the baby and also speeds tummy tightening. For baby, breastfeeding provides comfort along with the perfect food. Breast milk provides nutrients and immune antibodies that commercial formula simply cannot compete with. For more, please see pg. 143-148 of this book.

- **to ease baby's delicate digestion:** avoid these foods when nursing: high sulfur vegetables like broccoli, cauliflower, garlic and onions which increase gas and restlessness in your newborn. Chocolate, fatty dairy foods, eggs, nuts and soy may also trigger allergies in your baby.

- **for infected breasts (look for pain, redness, swelling on the infected breast, and low grade fever):** 500mg vitamin C every 3 hours, 400IU vitamin E, and beta-carotene 10,000IU daily; chlorophyll from green salads, green drinks, or green supplements—Crystal Star Energy Green Renewal™ or Green Foods Green Magma. For mastitis—redness, fever, flu-like symptoms—consult a health care professional.

- **for caked or crusted breasts:** simmer elder flowers in oil and rub on breasts. Wheat germ oil, almond oil and cocoa butter are also effective, or use Earth Mama Angel Baby Natural Nipple butter.

- **for yeast infection of the breast:** eat yogurt daily and keep nipples clean and dry. Apply acidophilus powder paste daily. Paint on a solution of gentian violet, available through many pharmacists but be aware it can stain clothing (highly effective, short term use only, excessive use of gentian violet may cause mouth sores in babies). Take garlic caps or Wakunaga Kyolic caps daily. Nature's Path Ionized Silver-Lyte, or Nutricology Prolive (Olive leaf extract) provide relief for stubborn cases. Ask your healthcare professional first if pregnant or nursing.

- **for engorged breasts during nursing:** for prevention, nurse your baby every 2 or 3 hours in the first few days after birth. For relief, lie on your back to drain excess flow. Allow baby to nurse until breasts soften (if possible), and pump breasts if you miss a feeding. Apply ice bags to your breasts to relieve pain; or use a marshmallow root fomentation with 1/2 cup powder to 1 qt. water. Simmer 10 minutes. Soak a cloth in mix and apply to breast. Try Motherlove Breast Compress or Earth Mama Angel Baby Booby Tubes.

- **for low milk flow:** drink plenty of pure water, juices and herbal broths. Continue taking your prenatal vitamins and don't begin any drastic weight loss plan. The baby is still dependent on you for its nutrient supply. See "About Breastfeeding" on pg. 143-148. Many herbs have galactagogue properties (promoting milk flow), see pg. 108-110 for the herbs and products you can rely on for results.

- **for sagging breasts after weaning:** MagiaBella Bust Support or Baywood Breast Maximizing Lotion.

Colds

Pregnant women catch colds just like everyone else, but over-the counter drugs for congestion relief and antibiotics are not a good choice during pregnancy. They tend to drive the infection deeper and some can affect the baby. Natural therapies, in contrast, help restore immune strength while reducing symptoms.

For cold prevention, avoid contact with people who are sick, practice relaxation therapies to cut pregnancy-related stress, and focus on a balanced, whole foods diet. For acute colds, avoid antibiotics and over the counter drugs unless your doctor is absolutely sure they're necessary. Try homemade chicken soup instead; it works wonders! Add garlic and onions for anti-infective qualities.

Eat vitamin C foods for immune response: citrus fruits and juices, broccoli, greens, papaya, potatoes, tomatoes. Vitamin C chewables help reduce runny nose and allergy eye symptoms. AMERICAN HEALTH VITAMIN C ACEROLA PLUS (highly effective). Elderberry syrup (use berry only-not the root) is a specific for flu. Try a very dilute eucalyptus or tea tree steam treatment to ease coughing or respiratory symptoms. Just add a few drops to a vaporizer and breathe in for relief. Have hot herbal teas, especially peppermint or ginger to promote sweating, and miso or nutritional yeast broths often. Use MAITAKE PRODUCTS MAITAKE D-FRACTION extract as directed to rebuild immune strength.

Constipation

Hormonal changes during pregnancy slow down the digestive system and often cause constipation. Commercial iron supplements used during pregnancy can be constipating, too.

Add fiber fruits, like prunes, figs and apples, and 1 tbsp. ground flax seeds to your daily diet. Increase your fluid intake to 10 or 12 cups of water or other non-caffeinated drinks daily. Regular exercise, especially yoga, can help. Make your own slippery elm anti-constipation hot cereal. Take a small handful of slippery elm (inner bark), and cover in a pot with rice milk. Warm until it reaches the consistency of oatmeal. Top with a little cinnamon and honey. (Bran cereal also works well.) Try oat bran fiber as a bulking agent and JARROW JARRO-DOPHILUS for friendly bacteria support. Homeopathic Nux Vomica tabs 6X three times daily (especially for constipation with nausea). Red clover infusion is a specific. Kelp tabs help lubricate and move the bowels without risks.

Diabetes (Gestational)

Pregnancy hormones can block the action of insulin, leading to insulin resistance and high blood sugar levels. Gestational diabetes affects 4% of pregnant women, usually develops in the fifth or sixth month of pregnancy, and is more common in women over 35. A blood test performed in the 6th month of pregnancy will detect gestational diabetes. If sugar levels are left uncontrolled, the baby is at higher risk for having low blood sugar, jaundice, and being born overweight. Gestational diabetes usually goes away when baby is born, but it increases risk for type 2 diabetes later in life.

Normalize high blood sugar swings with a low fat, high fiber diet and moderate exercise. Avoid sweets like candy, cake, ice cream and cookies. If you crave sweets, have an apple or pear, they're high in fiber to help eliminate excess sugar in the blood. Eat smaller meals to reduce the workload on your pancreas. Add a few pinches of cinnamon to herbal teas or hot cereal for sugar regulation help. HERBAL ANSWER'S ALOE FORCE juice (aloin-free) helps balance blood sugar levels and can be used by pregnant women. Consider MAITAKE PRODUCTS MAITAKE SX-FRACTION to reduce insulin resistance. If you're planning for another baby in the future: Avoid gaining extra weight between your pregnancies. It can be a significant risk factor for gestational diabetes.

False Labor

Braxton Hicks contractions are relatively common during late pregnancy. Catnip tea or red raspberry tea will help. See also MISCARRIAGE pg. 66-73 in this book.

How can you tell false labor from real labor?

False labor symptoms from the American Pregnancy Association - www.americanpregnancy.org:

- Braxton Hicks contractions are unpredictable and irregular (occurring in intervals of ten minutes, then two minutes, then six minutes, etc.)

- there is no labor progression over time

- usually no bloody show (see true labor symptoms for more on bloody show)

- membranes will not rupture (water breaking)

- contractions feel like abdominal tightening

- a change in position or activity causes contractions to stop or slow down

About a month before you give birth, your body will give you signs that it's becoming ready. Some women will notice a burst of energy with the desire to prepare things around the house, like having baby's room very organized, freezing extra food or cleaning out dirty cupboards. One of the biggest signs that you're becoming ready is when your baby drops lower into your pelvis, called "lightening." Women report this can make breathing and digestion easier, but urination even more frequent!

True labor symptoms from the American Pregnancy Association - www.americanpregnancy.org:

- contractions follow a regular pattern, occurring closer together as labor progresses. Use a stopwatch to time your contractions.

- contractions last longer than 30 seconds at the onset and become progressively longer (up to a minute) and more intense.

- presence of bloody show. Bloody show is the presence of a small amount of blood or pinkish discharge that usually occurs around the 40th week of pregnancy. Large amounts of blood are not normal and could be a sign of uterine hemorrhage. Seek medical help immediately.

- membranes will rupture (water breaking)

- pain begins high in the abdomen and radiates throughout your abdomen and lower back

- contractions persist and labor progresses regardless of changes in position or activity

Report any signs of false or true labor to your physician. A medical exam can tell you whether or not your cervix is dilated. Some lucky women may only feel pressure or back pain in early labor. Others will have intense, painful contractions. Some women's labors progress quickly while others labor much longer. Wherever you fall, take comfort in the fact that labor and childbirth are natural processes that your remarkable body was designed for. Take proper care and remind yourself that women all around the world have been giving birth for millennia.

Fatigue

Rising progesterone levels during pregnancy can lead to one of the worst pregnancy-related symptoms: fatigue. Fatigue is normally most severe during the first and third trimesters.

Take cat naps and frequent breaks whenever you can. Light exercise like yoga stretches and walking revive body energy. Try a green drink midday like CRYSTAL STAR ENERGY GREEN™ or ALL ONE MULTIPLE VITAMINS & MINERALS green phyto base instead of a sugary snack. Don't skip your prenatal vitamins. They can make all the difference for pregnancy-related fatigue. Get checked for anemia if fatigue is severe or long lasting.

Gas/Heartburn

Heartburn is a bothersome condition in the last trimester, and for women who are pregnant with multiples. Usually caused by increased pressure from the growing baby sitting under your stomach and because pregnancy hormones can cause over relaxation of the sphincter between the esophagus and stomach.

Sit up after meals and avoid fatty, fried foods and caffeine. Try eating smaller meals with plenty of fiber. Avoid drinking acidic juices like orange juice on an empty stomach. Try having a little yogurt or kefir instead. Fermented dairy foods can help neutralize an over-acid stomach. Take AMERICAN HEALTH PAPAYA CHEWABLES or papaya juice with a pinch of ginger (any kind) for gas relief. For gas after meals, try a weak tea with fennel, spearmint, peppermint or chamomile, or TRANSFORMATION DIGESTZYME. For fast relief of symptoms, consider EARTH MAMA ANGEL BABY HEARTBURN TEA (highly recommended). Try XLEAR SPRY xylitol chewing gum to fight heartburn. Xylitol also reduces your child's risk for cavities later!

Headache

Pregnant women may experience headaches caused by low blood sugar. Tension headaches are also common. Severe headaches in late pregnancy may be a sign of toxemia. Ask your physician.

Fight low blood sugar headaches by eating small meals throughout the day. Drink plenty of fluids to prevent dehydration, a common cause of blood vessel constriction. Use an ice pack on the base of your neck for relief. CRYSTAL STAR CALCIUM MAGNESIUM SOURCE™ caps helps relieve vascular spasms. Try a chamomile/lemon balm/catnip tea with a dropperful of scullcap extract for relief of tension headaches. MYGRASTICK by HEALTH FROM THE SUN works in a pinch.

Hemorrhoids

Increased pelvic floor pressure from pregnancy can lead to hemorrhoids—painful, swollen varicose veins of the rectum.

Add more fiber to your diet and see recommendations for Constipation on pg. 115 of this book. Don't strain during bowel movements. Apply: CRYSTAL STAR HEMR-EZE™ gel, or EARTH MAMA BOTTOM BALM with rosemary oil and St. John's wort, or MOTHERLOVE RHOID BALM (all highly recommended). Try keeping your choice of topical hemorrhoid treatments in the refrigerator for the best results. Cold temperatures constrict swollen veins.

Insomnia/Difficult Sleep

Insomnia and difficult sleep affect most pregnant women, particularly during the third trimester, as the baby begins to move more and trips to the bathroom become more frequent.

Have a leafy green salad at dinner time for natural nervine action from calcium and magnesium. Or, try CRYSTAL STAR CALCIUM MAGNESIUM SOURCE™ or FLORA CALCIUM MAGNESIUM liquid. Nervine herbs help, too; Add a dropperful of scullcap extract to a cup of chamomile or passionflowers tea. BACH RESCUE REMEDY drops gently help insomnia caused by anxiety within 20 minutes. A pregnancy body pillow can work wonders for comfort and support during the last trimester. Try different sizes and shapes to see what works best for you. Try deep breathing exercises, foot reflexology massage or a warm (not hot) bath before bed for relaxation.

Labor

4 million women give birth in America every year! Your body is uniquely designed for this experience. Prepare a birthing plan in advance. Working with a doula or midwife is highly recommended. See pg. 132 for more information on your birthing options.

- **While in early labor, eat, drink and walk when you feel like it.**
- **Hydrate with cool drinks or chew on ice chips** even if you feel nauseated.
- **Russian remedy:** Suck on fresh cranberries periodically to help stimulate thirst.
- **For nausea during labor,** take ginger or red raspberry tea, or miso broth, or ALACER EMERGEN-C with a little salt added to prevent dehydration.
- **For labor pain,** take crampbark extract, scullcap or St. John's wort extract in water.
- **Try homeopathic Gelsemium to reduce fear during childbirth.**
- **For nerve pain,** apply St. John's wort oil to temples and wrists; or use rosemary/ginger compresses.

- **For sleep during long labor:** use scullcap extract. (Scullcap may be used throughout labor for relaxation.)
- **Labor bodywork:** Changing positions helps (try squatting or kneeling); take short walks or get on hands and knees. Have a partner massage you to relieve back labor. Try a warm shower or bath ("aquadural") to ease pain and contractions. Midwives find this works especially well after a woman has dilated to 4-5 cm.
- **Biofeedback and massage** have documented success for reducing labor pain.
- **Acupressure treatments** during labor reduce stress, pain and increase dilation. One of my personal friends used acupressure during her labor with good results.
- **Hypnosis** helps stop the flow of catecholamines, stress hormones that hinder the birthing process. For more information on HypBirth, check out *hypbirth.com* or call 818-248-0888.

Do you want to induce labor?

Women in very late pregnancy complain of lack of sleep, discomfort from pressure, increased hemorrhoids, urinary urgency or frequency, and a score of other pregnancy-related problems. It should be no surprise that natural means to induce labor are of great interest today. However, we don't recommend trying to induce labor before 40 weeks. After 40 weeks, it could be helpful to try the following methods. We've added a few old wives' tales here because the women we spoke to were so adamant that they worked.

Have sex. Having sex can stimulate contractions. Further, semen contains prostaglandins, which helps soften the cervix in preparation for labor. We've spoken to women who have used this approach with success. Try having your partner stimulate your nipples, too. Some women report that helps.

Walk around. Now is a good time to get a little exercise. Walking around can help position your baby and get you ready for labor. Try modified squats as you approach your due date. Squats help you prepare for the feeling of opening up during delivery. If squatting is too difficult, try a birthing ball (good results).

Try herbs, but don't go at it alone. Midwives report that small, frequent doses of black cohosh tincture (about 1 dropperful every hour) can help relax the cervix and uterine muscles. Blue cohosh is also used by midwives to induce labor with good results. But, to avoid risks to you and your baby, don't try these herbs on your own. We highly recommend you consult with an experienced midwife, doula or clinical herbalist before using herbs to induce labor. For your self-care, evening primrose oil helps soften the cervix. It won't start contractions, but can help prepare you for delivery. Dosage: 1300mg capsules 2x a day in the last 3 weeks of pregnancy.

Smoked oysters. Sounds weird, but one woman said it worked for 4 of her pregnancies! Our friend and colleague, Leah, was not so lucky when she tried smoked oysters to induce her labor as she reached full term with twin boys.

Prune juice. This is another old wives' tale, but a friend said it worked for her. In theory, prune juice has laxative properties that can help bring on your labor. Just don't overdo it or you might get really gassy.

Castor vegetable oil. Castor oil is a strong laxative that can bring on labor. In one study, women who received an oral dose of castor oil (60 mL- about 4 tbsp.) were more likely to go into labor within 24 hours than women who received no treatment. Castor oil is a much stronger laxative than prune juice, can cause emesis (vomiting) and is less forgiving to the palate. Our vote: Try only if desperate and with midwife guidance. Just 1 tbsp. may be enough. Rubbing a little castor oil on your belly and covering with a warm towel can also help induce labor if the cervix has softened.

Morning Sickness/Nausea/Vomiting

Morning sickness with nausea and vomiting is a problem for about half of all pregnant women. Experts now say morning sickness is actually a good indication of a healthy pregnancy outcome (women with morning sickness are less likely to miscarry). The cause of morning sickness is not well understood. During the first trimester, morning sickness may be Nature's way of protecting the tiny fetus from infectious organisms or toxic chemicals that may still be present in the mother's body. Dramatic hormone fluctuations play a role, too. Very severe cases may require medical intervention with intravenous fluids. Vitamin B6 injections are sometimes helpful.

Use homeopathic Ipecac, Nux vomica and Nat Mur, add vitamin B-6, 50mg 2x daily as soon as you find out you're pregnant to try and prevent morning sickness. Eat small meals. Focus on cold, plain foods. Avoid hot, spicy dishes. Drink fluids about 45 minutes before or after meals to help prevent vomiting. Choose foods that are slightly sour or salty to help replace minerals lost through vomiting. High fat dairy products aggravate morning sickness for many women. Watch cooking odors, too. They can trigger morning sickness relapses. Sip mint tea or EARTH MAMA ANGEL BABY MORNING WELLNESS tea, and eat rice crackers when queasy. Some experts report good results for curbing nausea with sauerkraut juice, or taking a little lemon juice in water before meals. Try AMERICAN HEALTH PAPAYA CHEWABLES to help curb nausea and stomach upset after meals.

Ginger works in clinical trials: 1 gram daily. Crystallized or pickled ginger, ginger syrup, ginger tea (add mint if you like) or ginger caps work just fine. My tester tried NEW CHAPTER GINGER WONDER SYRUP with good results for her first trimester morning sickness. Use in a tea or make your own homemade ginger ale. Also try: Acidophilus powder 1/4 tsp. 3x daily to rebalance the stomach and GI tract; a travel sickness wrist band to stimulate the acupressure point (Neiguan point) that reduces nausea. **Note:** Take your prenatal vitamins with food in the evening or whenever you are feeling your best to help shore up nutrients for the baby.

Miscarriage

Seek medical advice and see MISCARRIAGE page 66 for detailed information on natural therapies. Raspberry tea every hour with 1/4 tsp. ascorbate vitamin C powder added, and drops of hawthorn extract every hour is helpful for prevention and hemorrhage control.

Postpartum Depression

Postpartum depression is linked to dramatically shifting hormone levels and exhaustion after childbirth. Natural therapies help ease the "baby blues" along with support from loving friends and family. See pg. 150 for more information on postpartum depression.

Preterm Premature Rupture of Membranes (Pprom)

Preterm premature rupture of the membranes that occurs before the 37th week of pregnancy occurs in 2% of pregnancies. Premature rupture of membranes is a serious concern because it significantly increases risk of preterm labor and infections for the mother and baby (chorioamnionitis-placental infection). However, in some cases, what is defined as premature rupture of the membranes is more of a minor leak caused by a small tear in the membranes which sometimes heals over. If there is only minor leakage, bed rest can help a mom carry the baby longer, so his or her lungs will be better developed when born. Cigarette smoking, vaginal infections and membrane weakness all play a role in premature rupture of membranes. Check your risk factors. If your water breaks or you experience leakage before you're due, seek medical attention right away.

Vitamin C is a specific for prevention through its collagen enhancing activity. In a study conducted by the *National Institute of Perinatology*, expectant mothers in their 20th week were given 100mg of vitamin C. Premature rupturing of the membranes occurred in about 8% of these mothers versus 24% of the placebo group. Vitamin C helps maintain the integrity of the chorioamniotic membranes.

Shortness of Breath

In the first trimester, rising progesterone levels can temporarily cause shortness of breath. In the last trimester, symptoms can return as your growing baby exerts pressure on your diaphragm. Shortness of breath will not normally affect your child's oxygen supply. To reduce discomfort, try sitting up and standing to alleviate pressure on the diaphragm. Use pillows to prop up your body while sleeping. BACH FLOWERS RESCUE REMEDY alleviates anxiety.

Skin Problems

Hormonal changes, increases in blood volume, stretching skin and new allergies all present challenges to your skin during pregnancy. Pigmentation issues, itching skin, new moles, skin tags and pregnancy acne can be a problem.

Use a mild cleanser like YOANNA SKIN CARE CUCUMBER CLEANSER or MYCHELLE DERMACEUTICALS FRUIT ENZYME CLEANSER. To reduce discoloration patches, try YOANNA SKIN CARE CUCUMBER PEARL CREAM. Itching skin can be caused by an overtaxed liver, try a dandelion (root and leaf) or yellow dock tea 3 – 4 times a week for relief. Take an oatmeal bath for almost immediate relief of itching and skin rashes. For pregnancy mask (chloasma), avoid sun exposure; it worsens the condition. If you have pregnancy skin tags, schedule their removal with a dermatologist after you give birth.

Stretch Marks & Post Pregnancy Tummy Bulge

Stretch marks can be a pregnant woman's worst fear. Women long for the days when they could wear bikinis and baby-doll t-shirts. Stretch mark severity depends on genetics and nutrition. Pregnancy stretch marks tend to fade with time, and some women don't get them at all. Don't dwell if you do get them. Be proud of your hard work "growing" your little miracle. Almost all women will have a little tummy bulge after they give birth that may hang on for some time. Severe cases of diastasis, caused by the separation of the outermost abdominal muscles during pregnancy, can benefit from an exercise program, a lean plant based diet and thermogenic herbs. Plastic surgery works well as a last resort, but be aware of the risks.

Improve your chances by pacing your weight gain and eating plenty of collagen building vitamin C foods like broccoli, cauliflower, citrus fruits, greens, papaya and potatoes. Drink plenty of water throughout your pregnancy to prevent skin dehydration. Apply wheat germ, avocado, sesame oil, vitamin E, or A, D & E oil to make skin stretching easier. A comfrey-calendula beeswax salve also works well. Take vitamin C 500mg 2-3 times daily for collagen development. Highly recommended for stretch mark prevention: Earth Mama Angel Baby Stretch Oil, a high quality, absorbable herb-infused oil. Use on bellies, bottoms and breasts throughout pregnancy for best results, (used by Gwyneth Paltrow during her two pregnancies). Mother's Intuition Tummy Honey is another effective product (great for moms expecting multiples). Magia Bella Ultra-intensive Anti-stretch Mark Concentrate can help prevent stretch marks during the third trimester expansion.

For post pregnancy tummy bulge and weight loss: After you wean the baby, try Crystal Star Tummy Bulge Control™ caps with Calcium Magnesium Source™ caps. Pilates abdominal strengthening exercises can help you get back in shape. Julie Tupler's *Lose Your Mummy Tummy* is a great resource for dealing with post pregnancy diastasis. **Note:** Don't push yourself to lose your pregnancy weight gain too fast. Allow your body at least nine months to stabilize and return to your pre-pregnancy weight. Focus on a healthy plant-based diet and regular exercise to lose weight the healthy way.

Swollen Ankles

Mild to moderate ankle swelling in the last month of pregnancy is a normal response to pregnancy weight gain, increased blood volume and the third trimester expansion. In the weeks before you give birth, you may also notice some vaginal swelling. Don't worry. This is just a temporary response to increased pressure. If it persists or is painful, schedule a check up with your doctor. **Note:** Extreme swelling that affects the face and hands could be a sign of toxemia.

Keep legs elevated whenever possible. Have your partner massage your feet for relief. Use NATURE'S APOTHECARY BILBERRY extract in water. Dandelion leaf (extract or tea) replenishes key minerals while reducing leg and ankle swelling. EARTH MAMA ANGEL BABY HAPPY FEET foot soak with yarrow and rose petals. Leah's choice: peppermint foot cream applied before bed. For post partum swelling: Nettles or dandelion leaf tea (steep for 15 minutes) are gentler than medical diuretics or water pills and produce good results for ankle and leg swelling after a C-section.

Toxemia, Pre-eclampsia

Affecting 7% of pregnant women, toxemia is caused by liver malfunction, poor nutrition and disease. The liver cannot handle the increasing load of the progressing pregnancy. There is a marked reduction in blood flow to the placenta, kidneys and other organs. Severe cases result in liver and brain hemorrhage, convulsions and coma. Toxemia is indicated by extreme swelling, accompanied by high blood pressure, headaches, nausea and vomiting. Pregnancy hypertension is also common, but if kept under control presents minimal risk to mother and child.

Vegan women have less toxemia risk. Especially avoid red meat and excess refined salt. Supplementing with vitamin C 1000mg and E 400 IU daily also shows positive results for reducing pre-eclampsia in high risk women. Green drinks, like apple-alfalfa sprout-cucumber or GREEN FOODS GREEN MAGMA offer a "chlorophyll clean out." Add dandelion greens as a mild diuretic to the diet 3-4 times weekly. Hawthorn extract helps normalize blood pressure. Use diluted in warm water. Add vitamin C 500mg every 3 to 4 hours, 10,000IU beta-carotene, bilberry extract in water, and B Complex 50mg daily. Iodine therapy via daily kelp tablets produces good results. Researchers from the University of Columbia find that supplementing with 650mg of calcium and/or 450 linoleic acid helps prevent pre-eclampsia for high risk women.

Uterine Hemorrhaging

During and after delivery, excess bleeding is a childbirth emergency that requires medical attention. Seek professional help immediately!

Astringent herbs can be helpful to curtail bleeding after delivery. Take bayberry/cayenne capsules. Take bilberry extract daily for tissue integrity. Use dong quai tea to normalize uterine contractions. For post-partum bleeding, consider shepherd's purse, false unicorn, nettles tea or an infusion of yarrow. Use under the care of a clinical herbalist.

Varicose Veins

An expanding uterus puts pressure on the inferior vena cava (a large vein that carries blood from the lower half of the body into the heart). This significantly increases pressure in the leg veins and the probability of developing varicose veins. Increased blood volume during pregnancy adds to the problem. Women who are overweight, have a family history of varicose veins or who are carrying multiples are at a higher risk. **Important:** Don't ever massage varicosities. Clotted blood could lead to a serious embolism.

Take vitamin C 500mg with bioflavonoids, 3 daily; or bilberry or hawthorn extract 2x daily in water; or butcher's broom tea daily (also helpful for leg cramps during pregnancy). Try daily inversions on a slant board. NATURAL BALANCE GREAT LEGS reduces leg heaviness and varicose veins (ask your health care provider first). Try a witch hazel/comfrey lf. compress for relief of vulvar varicosities. Take CRYSTAL STAR VARI-VEIN™ caps for relief of spider veins after you give birth. For very dark spider veins, sclerotherapy (saline injections) are useful after you give birth.

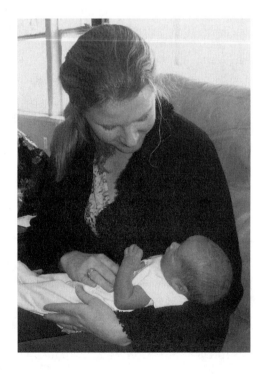

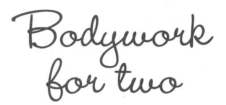

Chapter Twelve

E xercise eases pregnancy symptoms like insomnia, constipation and indigestion, and helps prepare your body for the high demands of labor and caring for an infant. A study in *Medical Science Sports and Exercise* reveals that women who exercised in early pregnancy experienced fewer discomforts in later term pregnancy. Exercise, along with a balanced diet, can even help prevent gestational diabetes.

It may take you some time to find the right kind of exercise for you. Exercising at a mild to moderate level, but not to exhaustion is advised. Some exercise is better than none, so even a short walk while running a few errands is helpful. Therapeutic bodywork like massage is another great choice for mild pregnancy swelling and discomfort. **Note:** If you have a high risk pregnancy, ask your ob-gyn what exercises are right for you.

1. **Strive for mild daily exercise**, such as a brisk walk for fresh air, more tissue oxygen and blood circulation. Light aerobic exercise, walking and dancing are usually well tolerated. Abdominal exercises like pelvic tilts (not during the last trimester) can facilitate a faster labor and help prevent post pregnancy tummy bulge. Water exercises and swimming are especially forgiving to pregnant bodies. Avoid activities like rollerblading, skiing and biking where a fall could injure you or the baby. Weight training or resistance activities should also be avoided.

2. **Take an early morning, or half hour sun bath** when possible for vitamin D, calcium absorption and bone growth.

3. **Consciously set aside one stress-free time for relaxation every day.** Yoga stretches (enrolling in a prenatal yoga class is highly recommended) and pregnancy massage are especially helpful. The baby will know, thrive, and be more relaxed itself. See "Prenatal yoga" below for detailed information.

4. **If you practice reflexology,** do not press the acupressure point just above the ankle on the inside of the leg. It can start contractions.

5. **Rub cocoa butter, vitamin E oil, wheat germ oil or EARTH MAMA ANGEL BABY STRETCH OIL on the stomach** and around the vaginal opening every night to make stretching easier and the skin more elastic during delivery. Many women swear that it makes an enormous difference. Gently stretch perineal tissues with your fingers to prepare for the birthing experience. Some women report that regular perineal massage eases childbirth pain and may help a woman avoid an episiotomy. See pg. 130 for more on perineal massage.

6. **Get adequate sleep.** Body energy turns inward during sleep for repair, restoration and fetal growth.

Prenatal Yoga - Perfect For Moms-to-Be

Prenatal yoga classes are highly popular today and are available in many parts of the country. Yoga helps you stay in shape while improving flexibility, posture and balance as your pregnancy progresses. Yoga practice relies on deep breathing techniques for enhanced relaxation and concentration, a major benefit for laboring moms. Deep breathing also helps your body relax instead of tense up, allowing for easier childbirths with less fear and pain. Modified squats increase circulation to the pelvic floor, and allow a woman to get comfortable with the feeling of opening up she will experience during childbirth. Prenatal yoga classes are also a great way to connect with other pregnant women, and share experiences.

Remember to breath through all your stretches as your instructor advises. Don't overdo it though. As your belly grows, some yoga poses may be difficult to maintain. Ease into challenging poses and skip ones that cause pain or discomfort. Inversion poses, belly twists and jumping moves are not recommended. Further, Bikram yoga in a heated room is too strenuous during pregnancy.

Prenatal yoga practice changes from trimester to trimester. During the first trimester, nausea from morning sickness, fatigue and fear of miscarriage mean many women avoid exercise all together, even though light exercise can be beneficial. During the second trimester, women have usually adjusted to the change, and moderate weight gain is not yet too cumbersome for their flexibility and posture during yoga poses. During the last trimester, modifications on poses and props often become necessary. For example, propping the head and chest up can ease shortness of breath from belly expansion and reduce pain from compression of the vena cava, (a large vein that carries blood from the lower half of the body into the heart). Experiment with the postures and breathing techniques that work best for you. Prenatal yoga is wonderful bodywork therapy for the stresses of pregnancy and childbirth, and the demands of life with baby later.

To find a yoga class or studio near you, visit *www.yoga.com* or call your local gyms and ask about prenatal yoga classes.

Massage away the aches and pains of pregnancy

Massage therapy is especially beneficial during pregnancy. Today more and more women are using massage to ease the aches and pains of pregnancy, and facilitate easier childbirth.

Some of massage's benefits during pregnancy

Helps release toxins and wastes that overload the circulatory and lymphatic systems, and contribute to fatigue and overall body sluggishness in the mother-to-be.

Acts as a mood elevator for pregnancy-related depression and anxiety. Stress-reducing activity of massage usually means deeper sleep for moms-to-be and more balanced blood pressure.

Significantly increases circulation, allowing more oxygen and nutrients to reach the systems of both mother and child for more vibrant health.

Increases the flexibility of muscles, a definite asset for the birthing experience.

Stimulates glandular secretions to balance hormone levels.

Reduces back pain, edema, leg cramps and swollen ankles caused by weight gain and body changes.

Light lower back massage (near the kidneys) promotes easier bowel movements for pregnant women with constipation. (If you get backaches when you're constipated, your transverse colon is probably blocked up by impacted wastes.)

May help reduce stretch marks and improve skin elasticity.

Note: There are some pregnant women who should seek advice from a health professional before undergoing massage. Check the following list for risk factors that may apply to you:

- pregnant women at risk for miscarriage
- pregnant women with cancers or tumors
- pregnant women with infectious illness
- pregnant women at risk for early labor
- pregnant women with pre-eclampsia (toxemia)
- pregnant women with gestational diabetes
- pregnant women with placental disorders
- pregnant women with heart disease, high blood pressure or kidney disease

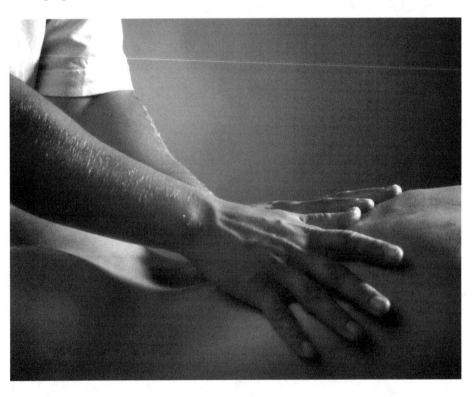

Perineal Massage: Is it a viable option?

Perineal massage is practiced by midwives and pregnant women all over the country with good results. Some women find they experience less stinging during childbirth after using this technique. Others report that they were able to avoid tears or an episiotomy after perineal massage treatments.

Perineal massage is normally practiced in the last six weeks of pregnancy to prepare the perineal tissues for the stretching of childbirth. The perineal tissues (between the vaginal opening and the anus) are gently massaged and stretched manually by the midwife, partner or the pregnant women herself. Some studies have disputed the benefits of this technique. One study suggests it is most helpful for women over 30. Ask your midwife, birth attendant or pregnancy massage therapist about the best techniques to try.

Three other techniques help prepare the vaginal and perineal tissues for childbirth:

1. **Apply hot compresses** regularly to help relax vaginal and perineal tissues for easier childbirth.

2. **Rub cocoa butter, vitamin E oil or wheat germ oil** on the stomach and around vaginal opening and perineum each night to make stretching easier and skin more elastic.

3. **Practice Kegel exercises** regularly to strengthen pelvic floor muscles.

How to practice Pelvic Floor Exercises (Kegels)

First, identify your pelvic muscles by stopping and starting your urine flow when you are using the bathroom. After you've identified them, practice tightening and releasing these muscles often throughout the day. Pregnant women should strive to do 25 repetitions of Kegels a few times each day. Women with a history of prolapses or incontinence may benefit from doing more. Practicing Kegels strengthens the pelvic floor for an easier labor and even reduces risk of incontinence after you give birth.

Chapter Thirteen

It's getting to be time

Hospitals, Midwifery, & Home and Water Birthing: What's the right choice for you?

Where to have your baby is an important decision for expectant parents. Hospitals offer the convenience of having medical professionals equipped to handle emergencies with you every step of the way, medications to ease labor pain, and neonatal care units for your baby if he (or she) needs help acclimating to his new world. Some hospitals offer birthing suites for laboring women with a home-like atmosphere, but with medical care.

Home and water births, assisted by a qualified midwife, are traditionally favored in the natural healing community as a less stressful environment for the mom and for the baby, particularly if there are no medical complications. Home births were the norm in the U.S. prior to the 20th century, but have since been a source of controversy because of safety concerns of risks to mother and child. You may have heard about a large study published in 2002 in *Obstetrics and Gynecology* which blasted home births for having twice the risk of infant mortality and other complications. Since then, this study has been criticized for major design and interpretation flaws. In fact, evidence from at least 10 studies suggests that attended, planned home births for normal pregnancies are as safe or safer than hospital births.

We've known women who opted for home or water births with great results, reporting their children attained long lasting benefits from entering the world gently and naturally. Unnecessary medical interventions are largely avoided with water or home birthing, and the couple retains a sense of control over the process. For instance, warm compresses are generally used to ease the child's passage, reducing the need for episiotomy. See pg. 137 for more on medical interventions during childbirth.

We've also known many women who have had hospital births and felt reassured from the constant support of the staff and the availability of Neonatal Intensive Care Units (NICU) to help care for their newborns. Birthing centers are another option for laboring women which offer a personal, family setting where the woman takes charge of her labor and birthing experience with help from a birth attendant or midwife. At birth centers, mother and child are never separated during routine exams. Birth centers are also set up to deal with transfers to the hospital.

Ultimately, where to have a child is a personal decision that both partners should make together with careful thought and preparation. Whatever your choice, be sure to prepare your birthing plan in advance, and try to be flexible.

Who to have in attendance for the birth of your child is another big question to answer before you go into labor. In times past, expectant fathers sat around in hospital waiting rooms or at home by the phone for news of the delivery after their wives went into labor. Times have definitely changed! Today, expectant fathers are encouraged to attend child birth education classes and play an active role in supporting the birth process for women.

If the woman is single, there are other good options for childbirthing support. Family members or caring friends can provide wonderful support. Many married women opt to have family members or friends present in addition to their husbands. If you're already pregnant, you may be considering care from a midwife or doula. A direct-entry or traditional midwife is a person (usually a woman) who has been formerly trained and certified or licensed (depending on your state) for assisting home births. (**Note:** Some midwives receive their training through apprenticeship under other experienced midwives.) A doula is a person who supports, comforts and coaches the women throughout labor and childbirth. A doula is generally trained and certified through midwifery schools, and acts to support a woman in her childbirth decisions.

An obstetrician specializes in pregnancy care and hospital delivery. He or she will have extensive training on how to handle a normal natural childbirth, complicated childbirth or the need for cesarean section. If you are concerned about your childbirth, want access to pain medications and medical interventions, have pregnancy complications or risk factors, a hospital delivery with an obstetrician may be the right choice for you. Nurse-midwives, who first receive formal training as registered nurses and then specialize in midwifery care, are also available in most hospitals. Many hospitals also offer doula referrals for childbirthing assistance.

We highly recommend taking advantage of your choice of childbirth specialists during your labor wherever you give birth. Interviewing potential midwives and doulas, and having a discussion with your obstetrician prior to the birthing can help to make sure all of your questions and concerns have been addressed up front.

Resources to learn more:

To find a midwife, visit the Midwives Alliance of North America or the web: *www.mana.org* or call 888-923-MANA (6262). It is important to note that in some states, the services provided by midwives are illegal. *Mana.org* offers a detailed state by state chart to check on the status of your state.

To find a qualified doula, visit Doulas of North America on the web: *www.dona.org* or call 888-788-DONA (3662).

Considering a Water Birth?

There are benefits to birthing in water

Water birthing has been around for centuries. Ancient Egyptian women delivered babies who were destined to become royalty by water birth. Women from indigenous tribes around the world have traditionally entered the shallow ocean or river waters to help ease labor pain and delivery. Water births are still widely practiced in Europe and are gaining popularity in the West. Laboring in water offers hydrotherapy benefits for mother and child. One Canadian study showed 100% of women who birthed in water used no pain medication. (Women who choose water birth are less likely to want drugs in any case.) Midwives say that birthing in water reduces pain by 20-80% for women. It is so effective that the term "aquadural" is popular among midwives as the natural alternative to an epidural.

Water creates a sense of weightlessness, so a laboring women's muscles don't have to work so hard at supporting her. Water also relaxes the pelvic floor muscles, decreasing birth canal injuries and the need for episiotomy. Birthing pain and pressure is reduced, and water birth labors tend to be shorter, provided a woman waits long enough before entering the water. (Most doulas suggest waiting until the cervix is dilated to 4-5 centimeters before entering the birthing pool. Entering the water prior to this may actually prolong labor.) Hot water from the birthing pool improves circulation to all the organs, especially the uterus, helping to protect the baby against fetal stress. Experts feel that transitioning from the womb into the world is easier for babies surrounded by warm water.

Many expectant moms worry their baby will attempt to breathe during a water birth. Barbara Harper, founder of Waterbirth International, reports this is highly unlikely. The trigger to start a newborn breathing is contact with air on its face. While the baby is submerged, it is still connected to the umbilical cord and receiving oxygen just as it did in the womb. Still, water birth attendants insist a women's legs and hips be completely immersed in water during the birth process. If she is partly out of water, the baby may breathe in both air and water, increasing risk for lung problems. (If the baby is in distress, a water birth may not be a good option. See below.) Other moms worry about the temperature of the water and how it might affect the baby. The temperature of the water is kept to about 98 degrees, normally well tolerated by mother and child. Higher temperatures can be exhausting for the mother and dangerous for the baby. During a water birth (or any birth), staying well hydrated is important, particularly if your labor is long lasting and you're in the water a long time.

We believe home births and water births attended by a qualified midwife can be a good option for uncomplicated pregnancies. Many new moms and dads who choose water or home births feel empowered by the calm and personal setting. Some insurance companies will cover home birth expenses with in-network providers, but others do not. Check to see what your insurance options are. If you choose to have a home or water birth, have a back up plan ready to go to a hospital with maternity and NICU units quickly if necessary. Unless you have a very experienced midwife and live within a few minutes ride to hospital, home births or water births are not the best choice for high risk pregnancies.

When a water or home birth is inappropriate

If a woman has pregnancy complications, is giving birth to multiples or has an infectious disease like herpes, a water or home birth may not be right. Here are some other child birth situations where a water birth may be inappropriate and medical intervention or guidance is advised.

Potential Meconium Aspiration: About 5-10% of babies pass some meconium (first feces) into the amniotic fluid before birth. If your water is stained green, yellowish or brownish when it breaks, a water birth may not be the best choice. Be aware that some infants pass meconium during birth, too. If a lot of meconium is passed into the water during early delivery, it should be removed quickly and the women should try to birth the child out of water to avoid accidental meconium aspiration. Slight meconium ingestion is fairly common and does not generally present a threat, but meconium aspiration can cause pneumonia or serious illness in the infant. If you suspect meconium aspiration in your new baby, seek medical attention promptly. When properly treated, meconium aspiration usually causes no long term damage to the lungs.

Fetal distress: If your baby is under great stress from a long labor, he or she may develop an irregular or rapid heartbeat and oxygen deprivation which requires medical intervention. If you choose a water or home birth, your midwife or doula should electronically monitor the baby's heartbeat when you first arrive to detect potential problems that would require a hospital delivery. After that, when you're in active labor, continue to monitor your baby's heartbeat periodically with a handheld device. If the baby becomes distressed during active labor, the woman should get out of the water for the birthing or go to a hospital right away.

Malpresentation: If your baby is breech in the Footling (feet first) or Franklin (bottom first) position, a water or home birth probably is not a good idea. The baby could go into distress and experience oxygen deprivation. In fact, some breech presentations may require C-section delivery. In Europe, water births are becoming more common with breech position and with multiples. In the U.S., aquatic birthing centers with adequate medical support to deal with potential emergencies are less common.

Shoulder Dystocia: Shoulder dystocia occurs when there is great difficulty delivering the shoulders after delivery of the head, and if not attended to, can be a childbirth emergency. It occurs most frequently in women who are having very large babies and in pregnant women with diabetes. If you have risk factors for shoulder dystocia, a water or home birth may not be right for you. Shoulder dystocia may be avoided by not pushing through a few contractions to allow the baby to rotate. Shoulder dystocia requires medical intervention to maneuver the child into a good position for delivery without injury. Sometimes if the mother moves on to all fours, the shoulders will dislodge by themselves.

Hospital Births - Medical Interventions to be Aware of During Labor

In today's world, we tend to think of childbirth as a medical procedure more than a natural process. While there is no doubt that modern medicine has certainly made childbirth safer for new moms and babies, childbirth is still a natural process and, for many women, is relatively uncomplicated. We truly believe most women know their bodies well and can respond to the demands of child labor by making their own internal and external adjustments. Allowing the laboring woman to retain control over her own birthing process and what she is most comfortable with the support of a doula, partner, ob-gyn or midwife greatly aid child delivery.

Having a birthing plan in advance is definitely suggested, but keep in mind that flexibility, both mental and physical, can help you avoid unreasonable expectations about labor or disappointments about how the birth went later. You may choose to have medical interventions during labor, but interventions are not always necessary or productive. A few examples.

Labor induction should be performed in less than 10% of women. Unless there is a clear medical reason to do so, I don't favor labor induction because if the drugs do not work, the woman will need to have a C-section. In addition, women we've spoken with report that induced contractions with the drug, Pitocin, are more painful than natural contractions. True labor contractions follow a natural rhythm and progression. Pitocin's contractions tend to be stronger without many breaks. However, there are cases where labor induction might be appropriate:

1. Your water breaks, but you don't experience contractions soon afterwards.

2. You have high blood pressure, diabetes or a serious infection.

3. The child is going into distress or you are well past your due date.

4. You are expecting multiples and are past your due date.

Breaking the bag of waters in early labor: The bag of waters is the amniotic fluid which surrounds your baby in utero. It serves as protection from bacteria or other infections that can travel up the birth canal. Women report that membranes rupturing feels like a trickle or like a gush of fluid. Your uterus may also feel heavier after your water breaks. About 15% of women experience their water breaking before going into labor. Most women have contractions first and then the bag of waters breaks shortly afterwards. Breaking the water bag in early labor does not usually provide any benefit and could increase chances of cord prolapses, fetal distress or possible skull injury.

Not allowing mothers to walk or move around, or eat while in early labor; restrictions on birthing position: Most hospitals allow and even encourage a laboring woman to walk around to ease pain and help position the child for birthing. Women in early labor need to keep up their strength, so if they're hungry and not too nauseated, they should be given the opportunity to eat and drink freely. Midwives often suggest both partners take a few minutes to eat before going to the hospital in early labor. (**Note:** If a Cesarean section is planned, a woman should avoid eating because food can interact with anesthesia medicine.) If you become dehydrated or complications arise during a long labor, a Hep lock might be a good choice to allow fluids or medication to be administered through a small plastic catheter inserted in a vein. A Hep lock allows mom to move around unencumbered by an IV bag and pole. Restrictions on birthing positions are another concern. Some women feel more comfortable giving birth while sitting up, squatting, on their hands and knees, or on their sides. Midwives report that giving birth while lying down actually increases your chances of vaginal tearing. Ask in advance about your options and consider different positions to see what works best for you.

Epidurals, IV pain medications: Some women know in advance they want to take advantage of opiate-based pain relievers or epidural analgesia during child labor and birth. We do not disparage any woman for making this choice. But, be aware that having an epidural or taking opiate-based pain relievers may slightly prolong your labor or increase your chances of having a forceps-assisted delivery. In addition, if you choose to use opiate-based drugs administered by an IV, your mobility may be very limited. A "light epidural" helps relieve pain, without causing complete loss of sensation. Talk to your ob-gyn in advance about your pain medication options. If you choose a natural childbirth without drugs, take advantage of childbirth education classes to learn breathing techniques that help during labor. Also, take advantage of the healing power of water during labor by taking a warm shower or bath to help relieve pain. Acupuncture and massage also work as effective pain relievers. See "labor" pg. 119 for more on natural pain relievers.

Episiotomies: Episiotomies are a surgical incision performed during childbirth to enlarge the birth canal by cutting the perineum (the muscle and tissue between the vagina and the anus). Having an episiotomy is often favored by obstetricians because it can help avoid uneven vaginal tears that are difficult to suture medically. However, women report that tears which occur naturally during childbirth actually heal faster than surgical cuts. Today, episiotomies are being performed at a much higher rate than necessary. Current statistics show a nationwide rate of 39%, even though most experts feel a rate of 10% is more appropriate.

In fact, research shows the majority of pregnant women get no benefit from having an episiotomy. An episiotomy may also lead to complications like painful intercourse after child delivery, prolonged healing time, infections, and problems with bowel control if the anal sphincter is accidentally damaged. If you're pregnant, talk to your doctor about your episiotomy preference during child labor. Perineal massage in the last month of pregnancy (see pg. 130 for more) and using warm compresses on the perineum during labor can reduce the need for an episiotomy.

What about Cesarean section (C-Section)?

A C-section is a surgical child delivery performed by cutting an incision into the abdomen and the uterus, where the baby and the placenta are then retrieved by surgeons. Surprisingly, some women are choosing C-section deliveries today because they want the convenience of "scheduling" childbirth. In addition, many women want to bypass the pain of labor and vaginal childbirth, and potential problems like vaginal tears, urinary or fecal incontinence or stretched tissues. Randomized studies on women who get elective C-sections are currently underway, but the results are not yet available.

Here's what we know so far: A C-section delivery is major surgery and is more complicated with a longer recovery time for the mother than a vaginal birth. Excessive blood loss and infection can result. It also presents drawbacks for the baby. A major benefit of vaginal delivery is that an newborn's respiratory system gets a boost as fluid in the lungs is squeezed out through the birth canal.

Babies delivered by C-section are more like to develop breathing problems like transient tachypnea (abnormally fast breathing) in the first few days after birth. C-section babies (even full term) are more likely to have respiratory distress requiring oxygen therapy. Most respiratory problems that occur after a C-section are transient in nature and can be managed with proper treatment. But, unless a C-section is medically necessary, as in the case of a placental disorder, a very large baby, breech presentation, or for a woman who has a very small pelvis, it puts unnecessary stress on mother and child.

The World Health Organization states that a C-section rate of over 15% is inappropriate. Today more than 1 in 4 babies are born through C-section. Vaginal delivery is still the preferred option for most women and their babies.

Here are a few things to keep in mind about vaginal delivery:

1. Urinary or fecal incontinence after pregnancy is often the result of having multiple babies in a row or having a poorly performed episiotomy. New research shows incontinence rates of menopausal women who have delivered vaginally and those who have never given birth are very similar. Incontinence risk from uncomplicated vaginal delivery has been overstated.

2. Most vaginal tears heal fast; a women may not tear at all during childbirth, especially if she has been stretching her perineal tissues during her pregnancy. Women who learn to relax their vaginal muscles also have reduced tearing problems during delivery. Having support from a doula or midwife during the birthing process also helps reduce your risk of having an episiotomy or vaginal tears.

3. While the uterus never shrinks back to its pre-pregnancy size, it does contract back to a normal, healthy size and vaginal muscles also recover quickly, especially if a woman has been practicing her Kegels.

What is a VBAC?

A VBAC is the attempt to have a vaginal birth after a previous C-section. Having a VBAC is often shunned by the medical community because of the risk of tearing the uterine scar from the previous C-section and the hospital's legal liability if there is a problem with the delivery. However, your doctor may be open to a VBAC birth, if you request it. Where to have the baby is another question to answer in advance because some hospitals have policies against allowing VBACs.

Is having a VBAC really that risky? A little history... A study published in the *New England Journal of Medicine* found that about 75% of women who attempted a VBAC were successful, and the mother and baby did just fine. Uterine ruptures occurred in fewer than 1% of these women who attempted a VBAC. In fact, the Department of Health and Human Services set a goal of a 37% rate of VBACs, because of concern that unnecessary C-sections take a heavy toll on pregnant women and health care resources. The VBAC rate peaked at 28% in 1996, but today has been reduced back to single digits. About 90% of women who have had a previous C-section will have another. A big problem: there are legal requirements to have a surgical team and anesthesiologist immediately (vs. readily) available during an attempted VBAC. Most hospitals simply cannot afford this, and do not want to take responsibility for a problematic VBAC outcome.

Ultimately, if you choose to have a VBAC, I think your wishes as a laboring woman should be respected. Discuss your choice with your doctor in advance and make sure there is no anti-VBAC policy at your chosen hospital. Medical monitoring of a VBAC birth is advised in the case that any complications arise. **Note:** Women who have multiple C-sections or who have vertical uterine scars are more likely to have VBAC complications than women who have had only one previous C-section and who have a horizontal or low uterine scar.

Twin deliveries

I've personally known women who have delivered twins vaginally without complications. Our friend and colleague, Leah, delivered her twin boys vaginally on Feb. 1, 2006 without complications. Still, twin deliveries are, by nature, more complicated than singleton births. There is a higher risk of going into premature labor with twins. In nearly half of all twin pregnancies, women go into premature labour (before 37 weeks). About one-third of them deliver early. (Thankfully, Leah did not.) Women pregnant with multiples should strive to reach 38 weeks, considered full-term in a twin pregnancy, to help avoid developmental problems and ensure a healthy birth weight. Bed rest may be recommended in the last trimester to help a woman pregnant with multiples carry to term.

Will I need to Have a C-section if I'm Having Twins?

The odds that a twin pregnancy will result in a C-section are about one-third, so there is still a good chance of delivering vaginally. However, most hospitals will have your twins delivered in a surgical room just in case. With twin pregnancies, the babies can be positioned in numerous ways: both head down (occurs in 40% of twin pregnancies, ideal for vaginal delivery), one head down and one breech (occurs in 30% of twin pregnancies, both babies may be delivered vaginally or one baby is born vaginally while the other is delivered through a C-section), or both breech (a C-section for both babies is likely). Still, some breech deliveries can be easier with twins due to the smaller size of babies. In addition, the second twin may change position after the birth of the first, making vaginal delivery easier. Your doctor can also move the breech baby internally or externally to help assist vaginal delivery.

How Long will I be in Labor with Twins?

Labor with twins is similar to that of singleton births in that it varies a great deal from woman to woman. Experience shows that the interval between the birth of twins is usually around 17 minutes. The first twin literally paves the way for the second, so the birth of the second baby is generally easier, although the woman still needs to push. Putting the first born child to the breast immediately after the birth can stimulate contractions to aid in the birth of the second twin. In cases where the umbilical cord prolapses or there is a placental abruption (the placenta tears away from the wall of the uterus) during delivery of the first baby, the second baby will need to be delivered by C-section. Working with a physician who specializes in twin pregnancy and delivery is recommended. Having a midwife or doula present can also greatly support your twin delivery process.

Chapter Fourteen

About breastfeeding

Mother's milk is best. There are so many good reasons to breastfeed your baby. Breastfeeding helps cement the bond between you and your baby. Newborns can only see 12 to 15 inches, about the distance between the mother's face and the nursing baby. Babies feel a sense of comfort and security being so close to mom. Tests show infants who are exposed to nursing pads soaked with breast milk instinctively turn to the one that smells familiar. Babies are able to distinguish their mother's milk through smell!

Breastfeeding is the best for baby's health, too. The baby who is breastfed receives Nature's "jump start" on immune response and gains health advantages that last a lifetime. We recommend feeding your baby breast milk for at least the first six months of life. Breastfeeding your baby for up to a year is highly recommended. Despite all the claims made for fortified formulas, nothing can take the place of breast milk. 80% of the cells in breast milk are macrophages, immune defense cells which fight bacteria, fungi and viruses. This helps protect breastfed babies from illnesses, like botulism, bronchitis, ear infections, flu, German measles, pneumonia and staph infections. Mother's milk also contains special antibodies to diseases that are present in the child's environment for added protection.

A child's immune system is not fully established at birth, and the antibodies in its mother's breast milk are critical. They fight early infections and create solid immune defenses that prevent the development of allergies.

The first thick, waxy colostrum is extremely high in protein, essential fatty acids needed for brain and nervous system development, and protective antibodies. Australian research confirms that children who are breastfed are 25% less likely to suffer from asthma or allergies later in life. Further, while babies have mixed results with formulas, they are never allergic to their mother's milk, although they could have a reaction to something in the mother's diet. Once removed, allergies subside. If you are unable to breastfeed long term, try to breastfeed for at least the first month to ensure that your child benefits from colostrum and critical nutrients that help establish strong immune defenses for later in life.

More good news about breastfeeding

Breastfed babies have lower risk of Crohn's disease, diabetes, eczema, lymphoma, obesity and SIDS (Sudden Infant Death Syndrome). Breastfed babies also have less colic. Breast milk is loaded with bifidobacteria, the beneficial micro-organisms that make up 99% of a healthy baby's intestinal flora—extremely important for protection against salmonella poisoning and other intestinal pathogens. Communicable diseases like diarrhea are reduced through breastfeeding. Mother's milk is also best for boosting and balancing your baby's fats. It contains the full range of EFAs needed for proper development of a child's central nervous system, brain and eyes.

The *Journal of Pediatrics* says that breastfeeding your baby may even make him or her smarter, giving your child an academic advantage! The determining factor seems to be the high content of DHA (docosahexaenoic acid) in breast milk, an essential fatty acid which comprises over 50% of the brain. DHA, vital to infant development, increases 3 to 5 times in the last trimester of pregnancy and triples again in the first 12 weeks of life. Studies show infants fed formulas supplemented with EFAs score significantly higher on Bayler Scales of Infant Development than infants who did not receive the EFAs from formulas or breast milk. Visual and brain development, and weight gain are all impacted positively. Formulas with algae-derived EFAs, rather than fish, were the most effective.

Over 60 countries have now approved supplementing baby formula with DHA and AA (Arachidonic acid) in order to more closely mimic mother's milk and ensure healthy brain development in babies, but breastfeeding is still the best for baby's health. Even with the recent addition of DHA and AA to formula, breast milk contains up to 160 fatty acids that are not added to infant formula!

Breastfeeding benefits new moms by increasing metabolism, allowing for faster weight loss after baby is born. Nursing also helps the uterus contract back to normal size. A study reported in the International Journal of Epidemiology shows women who breastfeed cut their breast cancer risk by nearly one-third! Like their moms, breastfed daughters have lower breast cancer rates when they grow up. A mother's ovarian cancer risk is reduced through breast feeding. In addition, as many new moms already know, breastfeeding can save your pocketbook. Infant formula can cost anywhere from $120-300 a month. There are rare cases when breastfeeding does present risks. Women infected with HIV can transmit the virus to the child through breastfeeding. In addition, women with breast cancer should only breastfeed from the unaffected breast and with guidance from her physician.

Q. I've heard you can't get pregnant when you breastfeed. What's the real story?

A. Women who breastfeed exclusively after childbirth may not ovulate again for up to 6 months, decreasing their chances of another pregnancy and allowing for more period-free time. Still, if you're breastfeeding and do not want to become pregnant, you should always use a back up contraception. Breastfeeding does not afford 100% protection! Stories passed from generation to generation confirms our breastfeeding grandmothers DID indeed get pregnant again while breastfeeding.

Are environmental chemicals present in your breastmilk?

It is true that chemicals from the environment are being leached into breast milk, the very foundation of human nutrition. In the U.S., nursing moms have 10 times higher levels of Polybrominated Diphenyl Ethers (PBDE), a family of flame retardants, in their breast milk than European women. Perchlorate, a chemical found in rocket fuel, now contaminates the drinking water supply of 35 states and is increasingly found in human breast milk and cow's milk. Perchlorate affects thyroid health by interfering with iodine absorption, and in pregnant women can lead to developmental problems in the fetus. In the United States, California and Maine have already acted to restrict the use of these chemicals. Human breast milk also contains hormone-disrupting PCBs and DDT, even in mothers who were born after the 1978 ban.

In spite of these findings, breast milk is still best. Researchers say that breastfeeding can reverse some of the damage caused by chemical exposure in the womb. Breastfed infants actually have a lower risk of childhood cancer and breast cancer, linked to chemical exposure. Further, switching to an organic, plant-based diet may help purify your breast milk. Research shows vegan mothers have less toxic chemicals in their breast milk than meat eaters.

Are you concerned your baby isn't getting enough milk?

New moms often worry if they will be able to produce enough milk for their babies. Relax. Almost all mothers are able to produce enough milk for one or even two babies.

Breastfeeding tips:

- **Avoid a drastic weight loss plan** when nursing because your baby is still dependent on you for a rich nutrient supply. Breastfeeding demands about 500 extra calories a day! Continue to take your prenatal vitamins to shore up important nutrients that may be lacking in your diet.

- **Your baby must have a good latch on your breast.** A nurse or lactation consultant can assist in helping your baby to latch on correctly.

- **Plan on nursing at least every 2 hours** or more during the day and every 3 hours at night even if you have to wake your baby up. The more your baby breastfeeds, the more milk you will produce to match baby's needs.

In rare cases, a new mother may not produce enough breast milk, usually because of poor mammary gland development or a hormonal imbalance. There are ways to tell if your baby isn't getting enough milk:

1. Poor weight gain (ask your pediatrician)

2.   Passing only small amounts of concentrated urine. If your baby urinates less than 6 times a day and the urine is yellow and strong smelling, he or she may not be getting enough breastmilk.

3.   Baby passes infrequent, small stools. A baby that is not getting enough breast milk may pass small, hard or green stools. Babies who are breastfed normally pass 2 – 3 large yellowish, watery stools every day.

For help with breastfeeding issues, we highly recommend consulting with a representative from La Leche League. For more information, visit *www.lalecheleague.org* on the web. You can use herbal formulas to encourage milk flow or weaning. For a list of herbs and high quality formulas, see page 108-110 of this book.

What's in that formula?

If there is simply no way to breastfeed your baby, cow's milk based formulas are an acceptable second choice. CARNATION GOOD START (for babies under six months) has a low allergy potential. Earth's Best is developing an organic baby formula to look for in the future. To learn more, visit *www.earthsbest.com*. Lactose-free formulas are another choice, well tolerated by sensitive or colicky babies.

Formula cautions:

Avoid formulas with high manganese. Infants are not able to absorb or excrete extra manganese. Early studies suggest children may experience learning or behavior problems from excess manganese. The FDA is now working towards reducing the manganese in infant formula to a minimum of 0.005 mg. of manganese a day.

Reconsider soy. Soy formulas are high in phytoestrogens which could affect the baby. Some research suggests that a soy-fed baby receives the equivalent of 3-5 birth control pills' worth of estrogen every day! Too much! If you can't breastfeed and your baby is allergic to regular cow's milk formula, try lactose-free or hypoallergenic brands. These are a better choice than soy, and are usually well tolerated.

Use pure water. Infants can be exposed to contaminants like arsenic, chlorine by products, lead, nitrates, pesticides, and solvents from tap water used to blend formula. Bacterial or parasitical contaminants are another problem, even in developed countries, which could lead to diarrheal illness or infectious disease in infants. When blending infant formula, use pure bottled water from uncontaminated sources. I've used and highly recommend PENTA bottled water. Another good option is to invest in a high quality water filter (AQUASANA makes a good one) to reduce tap water contaminants. To learn more about the safety of bottled water and municipal water supplies in your area, visit *www.nrdc.org/water/drinking/*

Always sterilize bottles before adding formula and feeding baby. Dirty bottles can make your baby very sick!

What about goat's milk?

If you can't breastfeed and your baby can't tolerate traditional or lactose-free formulas, a goat's milk formula may be an option you want to explore with your physician and nutritionist. A recent New Zealand study shows that babies who are fed goat's milk formula have growth rates comparable to babies who are fed cow's milk formula. Proteins in goat's milk are easier to digest than proteins in cow's milk, but these types of formulas should be used carefully and only for babies 6 months and older to avoid potential problems.

MEYENBERG'S pasteurized powdered goat's milk with Vitamin D and folic acid can be used in a homemade goat's milk formula recipe. *AskDrSears.com* offers a recipe for a nutritionally complete goat's milk formula that can be tried at home. Your doctor should also prescribe a multi-vitamin with iron if your baby is fed goat's milk formula.

A special note on using prescription drugs during pregnancy and nursing

Your baby needs your support for literally every developmental stage. Many of the prescription and over-the-counter medications you relied on before your pregnancy are no longer safe or appropriate after you conceive or when you're nursing. As a general rule, ask your doctor before using any drugs. In the first trimester, particularly when the fetus' tiny ears and eyes are forming and when the risk of miscarriage is at its highest, physicians consider drug therapy only as a last resort for most health problems.

Some specific examples… **The prescription drug Accutane** for acne is associated with very serious birth defects. It should never be used by a pregnant woman or a woman who could become pregnant. In addition, avoid antidepressants unless absolutely necessary. A new study shows the antidepressant Paxil is linked to twice as many major birth defects as other antidepressants! The research shows heart-related birth defects are rare but more common among women who took Paxil in early pregnancy.

Glaxo Smith Kline researchers estimate that the risk of cardiovascular defects is about one in 100 infants whose moms used Paxil in early pregnancy. There are other problems with using antidepressants during pregnancy. As newborns, many babies born to mothers on SSRI medications experience jittery nerves, irritability and startle easily. Used in the last trimester, infants may experience withdrawal symptoms from SSRI medications like trouble eating, body rigidity, and respiratory problems.

Over-the-counter medications like pain relievers, cold medicines and antihistamines can be dangerous during pregnancy, too. Ask your physician before using any over-the-counter medicines or prescription medications, even those you were taking before your pregnancy. Also, avoid alcohol, artificial sweeteners like aspartame, saccharin, and sucralose; aspirin, caffeine, harsh diuretics, Librium, MSG, Tetracycline, tobacco, Valium and X-rays. Even the amino acid L-Phenylalanine can adversely affect the nervous system of the unborn child. Especially stay away from recreational drugs—cocaine, PCP, marijuana, meth-amphetamines, quaaludes, heroin, and LSD. Your child may face addictive side effects and developmental disorders that could last a lifetime.

Everything you ingest affects your child and we only know a small amount about how chemical agents affect a developing fetus. Many gentle herbs and supportive nutrients can help you get through pregnancy-related health issues without great risks to your baby. Still, it is prudent to reduce standard dosage of any medication, orthodox or natural, to allow for the baby's tiny system. Consulting with a physician or qualified natural health practitioner is advised.

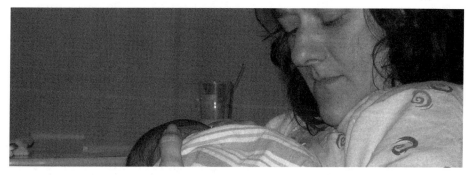

Chapter Fifteen

After your baby is born

Dealing with depression after childbirth: Can you lift Postpartum Depression (PPD) with herbs and special nutrients?

It's a problem that no one used to talk about: depression after childbirth. Postpartum depression (PPD) is gaining acceptance in the modern world. Thankfully, more and more women, even celebrities, are coming forward to share their experiences with depression and their recoveries. Postpartum depression affects about 1 in 10 new mothers. Less serious, mild depression (called the "baby blues") affects about 70 - 80% of all new mothers, and tends to disappear within 10 days of childbirth.

Physiologically, after pregnancy and childbirth, women are hit hard with a "hormone crash." Estrogen, progesterone and thyroid hormones decrease dramatically, often resulting in temporary depression. Major shifts in blood volume, blood pressure and immune response are other suspected triggers. Severe exhaustion—mental, physical and emotional—plays a role.

While physiological changes are involved in postpartum depression, lifestyle factors can't be ignored. Single mothers who don't have support in caring for their child are more likely to suffer from postpartum depression. New moms experiencing relationship or financial problems, or who are having problems breastfeeding are also more likely to become depressed after childbirth. Mothers who have multiple pregnancies close together or a history of depression or other mental illness are the hardest hit with severe cases of PPD.

Depression after childbirth leads to complex emotions—pain, despair, even concern for the welfare of the new baby. New moms often blame themselves and feel enormous guilt for feeling depressed after baby's arrival—a time when women are taught they should be happier than ever. If you're depressed after having a baby, give yourself permission to feel sad and seek professional help when you need it.

About postpartum psychosis

Postpartum psychosis is a disorder related to severe postpartum depression which requires medical attention. Women with a history of mental illness are at a higher risk. Look for these symptoms of postpartum psychosis, which usually occur in the first two weeks after childbirth: hallucinations, delusions, bizarre behavior, homicidal or suicidal thoughts. These symptoms shouldn't be ignored. Although it is a fairly rare condition (affecting 1 in 1,000 new mothers), postpartum psychosis consequences can be severe, and include child abuse, suicide and infanticide. Sadly, heart-wrenching cases like that of Andrea Yates, who killed all five of her children while in a delusional state shows just how serious postpartum psychosis can be. If you or your family suspects you're suffering from postpartum psychosis, we highly recommend immediate medical intervention from a qualified specialist. Appropriate treatment can help a new mom stabilize from these debilitating symptoms. Paramount importance should be placed on ensuring her safety and that of the child.

Do You Have Postpartum Depression?

Look for the following symptoms which may occur right after childbirth or in the subsequent 6 months. While mild PPD often resolves by itself, more serious cases may require medical monitoring.

• sadness; frequent, unexplained crying episodes

• mood swings, irritability

• low libido; fatigue that interferes with daily responsibilities

• difficulty concentrating, anxiety attacks or racing thoughts

• lack of appetite; or eating much more than usual

• sleeping more than usual; or recurring insomnia

- loss of interest in activities that you once enjoyed

- withdrawal from friends and family

- feelings of worthlessness, hopelessness or extreme guilt

- suicidal or homicidal thoughts (Seek medical attention right away! This is a sign of severe PPD and postpartum psychosis.)

Natural therapies lift your mood and nourish your body

1.   **Make sure your diet is as nutritious as possible** and get plenty of rest. Many doulas will help out with meal preparation, baby care and house work after the birth. Quick tip from experienced moms: Resist the urge to use the baby's nap time for housework. Sleep when the baby sleeps. The house may get a little messier, but rest is essential part of recovering from postpartum exhaustion and depression.

2.   **Make a post-partum herbal cordial** with 4 slices of dong quai root, 1/2 oz. false unicorn root, 1 handful nettles, 1/2 oz. St. John's wort extract, 1 handful motherwort herb, 1/2 oz. hawthorn berries, and 2 inch-long slices of fresh ginger. Steep herbs in 1 pint of brandy for 2 weeks, shaking daily. Strain and add a little honey if desired. Take 1 tsp. daily as a tonic dose. (Good results.) CRYSTAL STAR DEPRESS-EX™ caps are another premier choice for relief of the "baby blues."

3.   **Depression can be eased by B vitamins.** B vitamins assist with production of neurotransmitters that regulate mood like GABA, serotonin and dopamine. We recommend NATURE'S SECRET ULTIMATE B. New vegan mothers, in particular, may need to supplement with vitamin B12 to help shore up critical nutrients for breastfeeding.

4.   **Rebalance hormones.** Progesterone deficiency is a regular contributor to PPD. Consider progesterone balancing herbs like sarsaparilla root and wild yam, or an herbal formula like CRYSTAL STAR PRO-EST™ BALANCE roll on. Estrogen levels also drop after childbirth. An herbal estrogen balancer like dong quai/damiana extract can also perk up your mood and decrease depression. Add 2 tbsp. of sea vegetable to the daily diet for thyroid supporting iodine and energy support.

5.   **Supplement with the essential fatty acid, DHA (docohexaenoic acid).** Recent research from the National Institutes of Health reveals that

women with low DHA levels are more likely to suffer from postpartum depression. Consider New Chapter Supercritical DHA100, 1 daily.

6.   Homeopathy is a safe, non-toxic approach to PPD: Try Arnica for feelings of insecurity and depression after childbirth. Cimicifuga is for depression related to hormonal changes after childbirth. Cimicifuga especially helps the woman whose depression feels like a "dark cloud." Ignatia tabs work best for a sense of melancholy, along with feelings of grief, loss and depression.

7.   Aromatherapy lifts your mood and eases "baby blues"—Try a few drops of lavender, ylang ylang, vanilla or melissa (lemon balm) in an aromatherapy diffuser. Earth Mama Angel Baby Happy Mama spray is another good choice.

8.   You may feel tired, but make a concerted effort to exercise. Regular exercise is a natural anti-depressant that releases mood elevating endorphins. Walk with baby, or try swimming or aerobics. A friend bought exercise video tapes to do at home after her daughter was born. She lost her pregnancy weight much faster and felt so much better.

If you're suffering from the "baby blues" or postpartum depression, allow yourself time to recover. Postpartum depression generally goes away on its own in a few weeks to a few months after your baby is born. Natural therapies are an ideal choice for mild cases, avoiding side effects like agitation and weight gain that are common to drugs. However, if your symptoms are severe or chronic, seek medical treatment. Psychotherapy or treatment with antidepressant drugs may be necessary. Ask your physician before breastfeeding in these cases.

Preventing SIDS: Sudden Infant Death Syndrome

The topic of SIDS send shivers up and down the spines of new moms, but it's too important to ignore. And there is a lot of good news for concerned parents. There are easy ways to reduce SIDS risk, and keep your baby healthy and happy.

Every year, 3000 infants die of Sudden Infant Death Syndrome (SIDS) in the U.S. SIDS risk begins at about two weeks of age, and decreases after a child reaches 3 months. SIDS is very rare after the child reaches one year old. Just putting your baby on his back to sleep cuts SIDS risk in half because it helps prevent accidental suffocation. Today's pediatricians now recommend parents only place infants on their backs to sleep. Avoid loose blankets and soft bedding that could cause accidental suffocation. Don't bed share with other children in the house. Babies who share a bed with other children in the house are at a higher risk.

In addition, don't put hats on your baby on warm nights. A baby loses excess heat through the face and head. Covering these areas can cause babies to overheat, another SIDS risk factor according to European research. Wearable blankets are a safer choice.

Are toxic gases in mattresses to blame?

Toxic gases are thought to be involved in SIDS. Research done by Barry Richardson shows that toxic gases emerge from the interaction between common household fungi and chemicals like phosphorus, arsenic and antimony in baby mattresses. These gases may be a cause of suffocation. The risk of SIDS increases when mattresses are re-used on a second baby since by then, the fungus is well established. Using a chemical-free mattress cover like DR. D'S CRIB LIFE MATTRESS COVER may help reduce your child's SIDS risk. (Call 800-528-0559 or visit *www.johnleemd.com*.)

Other SIDS risk factors

- **Exposure to second-hand smoke** greatly increases the risk of SIDS because it reduces an infant's ability to withstand low oxygen levels if his face and head get covered. Even when a baby is merely in rooms where smoking occurs, the risk of SIDS can increase 800%!

- **Respiratory infections** may contribute to SIDS cases, particularly if the child has a fever and is put to sleep on the stomach.

- **A newly identified SIDS risk is a heart abnormality called a prolonged QT interval** which can be detected by an EKG and treated with up to 90% success rate.

- **Routinely feeding babies iron-fortified weaning foods** to prevent anemia may increase the risk of SIDS, according to the *British Medical Journal*.

- **The same H. pylori bacteria** linked to ulcers may be linked to SIDS. Scientists recommend avoiding transmitting adult saliva to very tiny babies to prevent H. pylori transmission.

- **Boys are known to be at higher risk** of dying from SIDS than girls. Boys are at higher risk, possibly due to their higher metabolism and propensity to overheat. The newest research suggests that male infants with the highest levels of testosterone are at the greatest risk. The research showed that infants who died from SIDS had 50%-120% higher testosterone levels in their blood than infants who died from other causes. Very high levels of testosterone may depress breathing during sleep, increasing SIDS risk. SIDS researchers believe that hormone monitoring in infants could some day help prevent SIDS in infants in this high risk category.

What else can you do to reduce SIDS risk?

First of all, try not to worry too much. SIDS is rare in children who sleep on their backs and who are not exposed to secondhand smoke. If you feel your child is at risk, a high tech T-shirt to monitor heartbeat and breathing is now available. Also, give your child a pacifier to use. Evidence from seven different studies suggests that babies who use pacifiers also have lower risk for SIDS. If your baby has a weak system, or poor lung tissue development (signs that he or she may be at risk for SIDS), consider vitamin C. Vitamin C has proved useful for reducing SIDS risk in numerous clinical studies. Breastmilk is higher in vitamin C than formula, especially if the mother takes a vitamin C supplement. I like AMERICAN HEALTH VITAMIN C chewables, taken as directed. Giving the child a weak ascorbate Vitamin C, or Ester C with bioflavonoid solution in water daily is another option that you may want to explore with your pediatrician. (The US RDA for vitamin C for infants is 35 mg.) In addition, if you're pregnant, low doses of carnitine (less than 100mg) during the last trimester can help protect the baby from SIDS.

Caring for baby, naturally

Caring for a new baby can feel like a daunting task, even for an experienced mom. In response, the baby industry is booming! There are literally hundreds of products to comfort and care for babies. And, there are hundreds of self-help books and websites with the "answers" to raising a healthy, happy baby. Through all of this, parents want to know what really works and what doesn't. The truth is every baby is different and what works for one may not work for another.

The best medicine for your baby is love, patience and thoughtful care. And there's no question that once bonding through holding and breastfeeding is established, pretty much nobody can comfort a baby better than Mom herself. New babies instinctively know their Moms, by smell and by sight. Dads, too, play a key role. Babies recognize Dad as a caregiver, and will usually be soothed and calmed through his loving touch and care. Having stated that, there are a few other tricks to keep baby feeling his best.

Natural baby care tips

Ask questions. If your baby is born at a hospital, ask questions, and pay special attention to the care and feeding tips you receive from the nurses. Nurses are highly experienced with babies and can give you a great deal of information on how to care for them. Consulting with a midwife or doula is highly recommended. A midwife or doula is highly schooled in caring for newborn, and is often experienced with breastfeeding issues. For more on breastfeeding, see pg. 143 of this book.

Diaper changes. Change your baby at least every 2 – 3 hours. Nothing is worse than leaving a baby in dirty diapers. Leaving your baby in a dirty diaper for an extended period of time is unsanitary and a great way for your baby to get a painful diaper rash. (See the following page for more.) New parents are often shocked to find out just how many diapers they will need. Babies need 10-12 diaper changes every day, at a cost of around $130 a month… double that if you have twins! If you're pregnant, stocking up on diapers in advance is a good idea. It will save you stress knowing you have enough diapers to last a week or two after baby is born. Remember, newborns need special newborn diapers. If you're at a high risk for premature birth, preemies need even smaller diapers. Cloth diapering is a great, environmentally sound option, but keep in mind the costs of a laundering system.

Tip: A baby needs your help to blow his nose. Use a nasal aspirator during diaper changes or before feedings if your baby seems stuffed up.

Bath time. Ask your nurse or doula how to bathe your baby. Many new parents are surprised to find out that a new baby doesn't need to be bathed every day. In fact, a light sponge bath is all that is recommended until the area around the umbilical cord heals. After that, a bath every few days with only the gentlest products is recommended. Bathing your baby more than this may dry out his sensitive skin. During a bath, don't forget to gently clean the creases under the arms, around the neck, behind the ears and in the diaper area. Wash your baby's fingers and toes, too. Baby's delicate skin does not need strong fragrances or harsh detergents. For baby, consider organic products with the gentlest of ingredients like NATRACARE BABY BATH or EARTH MAMA ANGEL BABY ANGEL BABY SHAMPOO & BODY WASH.

Bath safety: Don't ever leave a baby alone during bath time. And be careful with him in the bath. Newborns are very slippery! A special baby bathtub or plastic basin that fits inside the bathtub is recommended. If you're a mom of multiples, bathe your babies separately to avoid accidents. Keep the other baby (or babies) close to you while you're bathing the first one. Note: Don't keep the baby in the bath too long since they get cold quickly. If washing hair, save it for last, since babies lose heat through the head. Make sure the temperature of the room is warm, too.

Burping. Burping your child during feedings is key to supporting healthy digestion. Swallowed air in the stomach can cause fussiness and spitting up after feedings. Try to burp your baby when you switch breasts or after he consumes 1 – 2 ounces of formula, and, also, at the end of the feedings. Here are a few good techniques for burping:

- Lay the baby down on his stomach on your lap, and pat his back gently.
- Place your baby on your upper chest and shoulder, and pat his back gently
- Sit your baby on your lap or knee, holding his head and chin with one hand, and pat his back gently. Ask your nurse or midwife questions if you're unsure.

Trimming nails. You didn't think having a baby meant you would need manicurist skills, but, in some ways, you do. A baby's nails grow fast and they need to trimmed regularly so he doesn't scratch his face (ouch!). Try trimming your baby's nails when he is calm, but be very careful not to cut his sensitive skin. Another option is to carefully file down his nails while he sleeps.

Comforting a crying baby

Crying isn't usually a sign of serious illness. As long as your baby is eating well and gaining weight, does not have a fever or diarrhea, some crying is a normal part of baby life. By the time they reach 6 weeks, even babies that are not colicky cry one and a half to two and half hours per day. Babies that are defined as "colicky" cry more than three hours a day for three or more days a week.

Still, all that crying can be rattling to new parents and unnecessarily hard on your baby.

Tips to help new parents comfort a crying baby

If baby is very fussy, try swaddling him. Swaddling wraps the baby up very snugly in a blanket. Babies like the sensation of being wrapped up like they were in the womb. In a 2005 study published in the journal *Pediatrics*, swaddled babies were found to sleep longer and were less likely to wake up spontaneously than un-swaddled babies. Swaddling also helps prevent arm and leg flailing, and face scratching, major sources of irritation for new babies.

Here are helpful instructions on how to swaddle your baby from Elizabeth Rusch of *Plum* magazine, a special magazine for pregnant women over 35.

"Fold down the top right corner of a square blanket and make a triangle. Place the child on his back on the blanket with his head on the top fold. Fold a side corner across the baby and tuck it behind his opposite arm. Fold the bottom corner over the baby's feet and tuck it into the cross fold. Fold the second side corner across the baby, tucking extra material behind his back. You can also swaddle your baby just below the armpits so he can still use his arms." Childbirth education classes usually show parents how to properly swaddle a baby. Swaddling is so popular today that special swaddling blankets are available in most baby stores. We like Kiddopotamus SwaddleMe adjustable infant cotton wrap.

Make some white noise. Babies are exposed to a lot of white noise in the womb from mom's heartbeat and blood circulation (some say it's louder than a vacuum cleaner inside mom). But, when they finally arrive, we put them to sleep in quiet rooms! Some parents swear by taking a ride in the car, or turning on a room fan or vacuum cleaner to quiet a crying baby. Playing a CD with white noise sometimes helps, too. A baby blogger reports her baby liked the CD "For Crying out Loud." Babies love to hear mom and dad sing lullabies to them. Rocking baby and giving baby a pacifier are other good choices.

Hold baby on his side or stomach. Babies are often more calm when they are held on their stomachs or sides. But don't ever put a baby to sleep on his stomach.

Try a special baby swing to help calm your baby. But, keep in mind that not all babies like swings and the constant motion of the swing is not the best choice for sleep. Use the swing to calm your baby, then switch to the bassinet for sleep. FISHERPRICE portable baby swings work well.

Tip: A friend found her baby was the most calm when she was the closest to her. After a few weeks of struggling with the baby crying every time she put her down, she tried a baby sling to carry her close whenever possible. This gave the mother the flexibility of having her hands free to do chores and gave her baby the security of being close to her.

If you become very frustrated with a crying baby, take a short break by leaving the room for a few minutes. Ask friends and family for help when you need it. All that crying can really hurt your ears. A friend used ear plugs which allowed her to hold and care for her colicky baby with less stress on her own ear drums. **WARNING: Never shake a baby. It is child abuse.** Shaking a baby can cause serious injury, brain damage and even death. See the references section on pg. 171 for resources on child abuse prevention.

The benefits of infant massage

Infant massage has been practiced in other countries for centuries. In India, Africa and the Soviet Union, for example, massaging babies with special oils is part of a daily routine that begins soon after birth. Here in the U.S., massage schools are opening up to the idea of infant massage. Today, there are around 4,000 therapists that are trained to teach parents infant massage. Infant massage may some day be commonplace in the U.S. This is good news because giving your baby a therapeutic massage is a powerful healing technique!

Massage allows parents a new way to bond with their children, and has documented benefits for infant health and well being. A massage stimulates the vagus nerve which, in turn, stimulate peristalsis (rhythmic muscle contractions that move food through the digestive tract). A gentle belly massage supports your baby's immature digestive system by releasing trapped gas and stomach distension. Massage can also decrease teething pain, and relieve sinus and chest congestion.

After a therapeutic massage, infants sleep longer and appear to have longer periods of deep sleep. Other documented benefits of infant massage according to the Touch Research Institute:

- Newborn babies who have been exposed to cocaine in utero gain weight faster and are less stressed when they are massaged.
- Newborn babies who have been exposed to HIV gain more weight when they receive massage.
- Premature babies gain more weight, sleep better and are discharged from the hospital sooner when they receive massage.
- Babies massaged by mothers with post partum depression have lower levels of stress hormones, are less fussy and have more regular sleep/wake routines.
- Dads who massage their babies for 15 minutes daily have more positive interaction with them.
- Other reports suggest babies who are blind or deaf become more aware of their bodies through massage. Massaged babies with cerebral palsy may show more organized motor activity.

How to massage a baby

Always use a pure, cold pressed vegetable oil like grapeseed oil or EARTH MAMA ANGEL BABY HERBAL MASSAGE OIL when you massage your baby. (Avoid products with strong scents or synthetic ingredients. They are too harsh for baby's skin.) Allow the oil to warm up in the hands before the massage.

For the first weeks after birth, try a simple massage for 5 – 10 minutes. When baby gets a little older, progress to a 15 – 20 minute massage. A training session with a professional massage therapist experienced in infant massage is suggested.

Before you start: Pay attention to cues from your baby. If he becomes upset during the massage or begins to flail his arms or legs, discontinue the massage until he is calmer. Never massage a baby with skin infection or inflammation, unusual lump, fracture, or sun burn. Don't massage over an unhealed belly button.

A few basic tips to get you started

A nice way to introduce massage to your baby is by starting with gentle strokes on the legs. Place baby on his back on top of a blanket set on a flat surface and bring his knees to his chest by gently bending his legs. Hold the baby's position for a few seconds. Try this stretch one leg at a time, too. Use the opportunity to massage his legs, feet and toes.

Massage baby's shoulders. Start with your hands on the chest, massaging lightly up to his shoulders. Do this several times, taking the opportunity to also massage his chest, arms and hands with your fingertips and thumbs.

Massage baby's back by putting him on his stomach. (The soles of his feet should be facing you.) Gently massage from neck to the top of shoulders downward to the base of the spine. Use your fingertips to make little circles all over the back.

Abdominal massage with light pressure can decrease the severity and frequency of colic attacks. Look for signs of trapped gas like a tight, round stomach. Massage your baby's abdomen gently in a clockwise direction, without putting pressure on the diaphragm. Light abdominal massage stimulates the colon, releases trapped gas and helps push stool through the digestive system. A little crying is okay during this type of massage, but a lot of crying is counter productive. Discontinue the massage until baby is calmer.

Some babies like their faces to be massaged. Use circular thumb strokes from the forehead out to the temples. Apply light pressure with the thumbs or fingertips from the sides of the nose across the cheeks, too.

After the massage, swaddle the baby for a long, deep sleep.

For more information on infant massage, check out these helpful resources: *Infant Massage: A Handbook for Loving Parents* by Vimala Schneider McClure and *Baby Massage for Dummies* by Joanne Bagshaw and Ilene Fox.

Natural solutions for baby's special problems

Colds

A minor cold in a baby over three months is no reason to panic; even healthy babies have six colds or more before age 1. Infant colds generally last from three to ten days. **Look for:** fussy behavior, stuffy nose, dry cough and mild fever. (Flu symptoms are more serious and can include diarrhea and vomiting.) Frequent colds actually strengthen your baby's immune defenses. A baby has to develop immunity one cold at a time to the 200 or more different viruses that cause colds.

Preventive care: avoid contact with people who are sick. Wash your hands frequently. Clean the baby's toys and pacifiers often. For acute colds: Breastfeeding often is the best medicine here, providing rich nutrition and immune stimulating antibodies that help your child get better, naturally. To clear clogged passages, suction the baby's nose with a nasal aspirator often. Use XLEAR nasal wash as directed during diaper changes to lessen congestion. Using a humidifier with a few drops of eucalyptus oil in the baby's room can moisten the air and soothe his irritated mucous membranes. Offer dropperfuls of weak chamomile or catnip tea (antiviral).

In children less than three months, a cold may turn into more serious pneumonia or croup. Call your doctor at the first sign of sickness, particularly if the baby isn't wetting as many diapers, has thick eye or nasal discharge, has a bad cough, or is running a fever over 100.4 degrees. Serious symptoms that require immediate medial care include: difficultly breathing or lips and mouth area turning bluish; severe vomiting; coughing up blood stained mucous; or refusing to nurse or accept fluids.

Colic

About 25% of babies suffer from colic— meaning they fuss and scream for more than 3 hours a day for at least 3 days a week—no fun for new parents or for the baby. Intestinal gas, milk allergy and acid reflux are all thought to play a role, but they are not the only cause of colic. Colic generally goes away or is greatly reduced after three months, but problems with gas, allergies and reflux in babies persist much longer than that. Whatever the cause, there's no question that colic causes a lot of suffering for everyone. **Symptoms other than crying to look for:** Baby looks uncomfortable or in pain, the stomach may feel tight and round, and the baby may pass excessive gas.

New Theories on Colic

Harvey Karp, M.D., author of *The Happiest Baby on the Block*, theorizes that colicky babies are suffering from what he calls "the missing 4th trimester" in their first three months of life. During this time, he believes that babies are missing a calming reflex, which was stimulated by the sounds and comforts of the womb. After a few months, most babies adapt to the drastic change, develop new calming reflexes and cry less.

Try the calming techniques on pg. 157. They can work wonders. If you are nursing, watch your diet carefully. Sometimes mother's milk is acidic from stress or diet. Avoid cow's milk, cabbage, brussels sprouts, onions, garlic, yeasted breads, fried and fast foods. If nursing, consider a weak fennel seed tea or EARTH MAMA ANGEL BABY MILKMAID tea with added herbs to soothe baby's digestion. Avoid red meat, chocolate, alcohol, sugary foods and caffeine until the child's digestion improves.

Tried and true digestive remedy for colic: try WELLEMENTS GRIPE WATER with ginger and fennel. To promote healthy gastrointestinal flora, try NATREN LIFE START, 1/4 tsp. in water or formula as directed (also recommended for nursing moms).

Try Homeopathic remedies: Liquids are preferable, but you can use tablets with babies, too. Crush homeopathic tablets between two clean teaspoons and dissolve in 2 oz. of warm water. Use 1 teaspoon of the liquid as a full dose. Try Colocynthus, Chamomilla or HYLAND'S COLIC tabs. Effective weak teas include chamomile, peppermint and lemon balm (use just dropperfuls of lukewarm tea for infants). Never give honey to babies less than 1 year old. It has been linked to infant botulism. If the baby is four months old and colicky gas pains persist, offer them diluted papaya or apple juice, or small doses of papaya enzymes.

Bodywork: Give the baby a short morning sunbath for vitamin D. Try a gentle catnip enema once a week for gas release. Infant massage is specific for colic. Try the massage techniques on pg. 161. If symptoms don't resolve after a few months or are accompanied by frequent vomiting, it may be a sign of infant GERD (gastroesophageal reflux disease). Consult with a pediatric gastroenterologist if you suspect your child has GERD.

Cradle Cap

Cradle cap is a type of dermatitis found on the scalp in babies. It is a common problem, which is generally temporary and harmless. Still, if you see signs of cradle cap, treat it before it worsens or spreads. **Look for:** yellow, scaly skin patches on the scalp.

If you are nursing, avoid refined sugar which feeds bacteria and yeast. Use NATREN LIFESTART for infants to foster healthy flora. Massage scalp with vitamin E, olive oil or jojoba oil or EARTH MAMA ANGEL BABY BOTTOM BALM for 5 minutes. Leave on 30 minutes, then brush scalp with soft baby brush and shampoo with tea tree or aloe vera shampoo like NATRACARE BABY SHAMPOO or JASON LAVENDER 2-IN-1 SHAMPOO & BODY WASH. Repeat twice weekly. 10 day treatment: Apply cool comfrey root tea to infant's scalp or dry skin area, and let air dry in a warm room. Symptoms usually disappear. Cradle cap may be a biotin deficiency. Take biotin 1000mcg while nursing; the baby will receive the necessary amount through breast milk.

Diaper and Skin Rash

Diaper rash is a painful condition caused by sensitive skin, friction in areas where diaper elastic is too tight, and excess moisture. Look for: redness and irritation in skin folds around the inner thighs, buttocks and genitals. Stick to a diaper changing schedule every few hours. During changes, allow the baby's genitals to air dry for a few minutes. We recommend cloth diapers, or disposable diapers without harsh dyes or bleaches like TENDER CARE TUSHIES with real cotton to protect baby's sensitive skin. Note: Serious cases of diaper rash are often caused by overgrowth of candida yeast or bacteria (often occurs after a course of antibiotics for cold). Look for very red rash with raised borders and white scales.

Give plenty of water to help dilute urine acids. Wash baby with EARTH MAMA ANGEL BABY DIAPER RASH SOAP. Mix comfrey, goldenseal and arrowroot powders with aloe vera gel or calendula ointment and apply. Expose the child's bottom to indirect morning sunlight for 5-10 minutes for vitamin D nutrients (avoid direct sunlight in hot climates; the baby will get burned). Wash cloth diapers in water with 1 tsp. of tea tree oil (highly recommended for yeast overgrowth). **Topical applications work:** try MOTHERLOVE DIAPER RASH RELIEF; EARTH MAMA ANGEL BABY BOTTOM BALM; or JASON DIAPER RELIEF ointment. Homeopathic remedies help, too: SULFUR, RHUX TOX. Avoid petroleum jelly. Use talc-free powders like SKIN TREASURES BABY POWDER.

Ear infections

An ear infection may follow a bad cold, and can be very painful. Germs from the cold invade the middle ear and multiply, filling the space with infectious bacteria, pus and thick mucus. Around 2/3 of babies will have had one ear infection by the time they reach two. But antibiotics are not very effective for ear infection. 80% of kids who take antibiotics for ear infections don't get better any sooner! Look for signs like: child pulling at the ears, redness in the ears, fussiness, crying, problems sleeping and nasal congestion.

A new study shows kids who constantly suck pacifiers have 30% more ear infections than those who don't. Children exposed to cigarette smoke are more likely to suffer ear infections. For toddlers and older children, offer water, soups, herbal teas and diluted fruit juices. Also, try HERBS FOR KIDS ECHINACEA-GOLDENROOT to clear infection. For babies under 4 months, use a small amount of XLEAR NASAL WASH as directed during diaper changes. Topical ear support soothes pain and reduces inflammation: Use mullein essence, or MOTHERLOVE MULLEIN FLOWER ear oil, CRYSTAL STAR EAR DEFENSE, GAIA CHILDREN EAR DROPS, or garlic oil (antibacterial), or warm olive oil ear drops directly in the ear. Or mix vegetable glycerine and witch hazel, dip in cotton balls and gently insert in the ear to draw out infection. Studies reveal homeopathy reduces pain from ear infections. Consult a qualified homeopath to find out which remedy is right for your child.

Teething

Teething is a natural part of baby's development, but babies get more fussy as new teeth begin to cut through the gums.

A cold baby teether can really help. Watch babies that have teeth. They could puncture it. If baby has started eating solid foods, offer cold food like chunks of frozen bananas, but supervise closely to prevent choking (choking is most common in babies who have teeth). EARTH'S BEST

TEETHING BISCUITS are another good choice. Wash hands, and rub gums with a few drops of very diluted peppermint oil. Give weak catnip, fennel or peppermint tea to soothe. Licorice root powder (just a pinch) made into a paste soothes inflamed gums. **Effective products:** Use NOVEYA BABY TEETHING GEL or HERBS FOR KIDS GUM-OMILE OIL for teething. **Homeopathic remedies offer relief:** Boiron Camilia gel; HYLANDS TEETHING TABLETS. Avoid excessive use of teething gels with benzocaine; they may cause allergic reactions.

Thrush

Thrush is an overgrowth of candida yeast in the mouth. It is generally harmless, but can be a source of irritation or spread to the mother's nipples through breastfeeding (See pg. 114 for more). Look for a thick, white or yellowish coating on the tongue, or white or yellowish patches on the inside of the lips or cheeks. The child may stick the tongue out frequently, trying to get relief. Thrush is often caused by antibiotic use, and is more common in babies who sleep with a pacifier or bottle. Yeast infections can also be passed to the child during passage through the vaginal canal.

Make an acidophilus paste with water or breast milk and apply in the baby's mouth once a day (also apply on infected breasts). JARROW BABY'S JARRO-DOPHILUS is a good choice. Give the baby a weak ascorbate Vitamin C, or Ester C with bioflavonoid solution in water daily. (The US RDA for vitamin C for infants is 35 mg.) Ask your pediatrician.

You and your baby: a healthy lifestyle, a healthy future

Having a baby is life changing in every way. Congratulations on your little miracle and all the exciting changes and experiences that are soon to take place. Life will no doubt get very busy, but try not to forget the importance of your health—mind, body and spirit.

Keep your body healthy by eating nutritious foods that provide essential nutrients for your high energy lifestyle. Freezing healthy casseroles or soups in advance for the week is one option. Fresh foods are also highly nutritious and take little preparation. Grilled salmon (I use an indoor grill because they're fast), whole grains like bulgur or brown rice, and a fresh salad take less than an hour for preparation. When baby gets ready for solid food (between 4 and 6 months), try organic baby foods like EARTH'S BEST baby food or make your own fresh baby food. FRESH BABY SO EASY BABY FOOD KIT offers detailed instructions on how to make your own healthy baby food. When introducing solid foods, start your baby on greens early on to help him develop a healthy taste for them.

Pamper yourself when you get the chance. A new haircut, facial treatment or body wrap is a nice treat and it works wonders for your self-esteem. Don't skip on exercise, either. Regular exercise eases postpartum depression, helps tone your post pregnancy body, and protects your cardiovascular system from serious health problems. Most babies love long "walks" with Mom pushing their strollers. Bring warm blankets because babies lose heat quickly.

When time allows, keep your mind healthy with games and projects that challenge your creativity. Skip TV a few nights a week in favor of a favorite book, board game or craft project. Don't keep emotions bottled up, either. Share your feelings with good friends and family. Life with a baby can be trying at times, and it's okay to ask your spouse for some time for yourself or to have a good cry. Web forums and chat-rooms are a great place to get support from other new moms without leaving your baby at home with a sitter.

Try to make "alone time" with your spouse a priority. A date night once a week allows you both to reconnect romantically and remember why you decided to start a family in the first place. Caring friends and family are often glad to help out for a few hours.

We highly recommend relaxation therapies for the spirit like massage, yoga, tai chi, meditation or guided imagery after your baby is born. Just reading inspirational literature, sitting quietly or taking a walk in nature can help you relax and connect with your inner self. Finding your own spirituality and calm center reduces stress and helps you to provide a safe and happy environment for your baby to thrive.

We wish you the very best on the journey through parenthood. May your healthy lifestyle help pave the way for your dreams and your children's dreams to come true.

Love,
Sarah & Linda

Afterword by Leah Thomson-Vizcaino

Reflections on a new chapter of my life

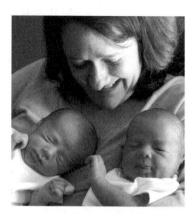

On Feb. 1, 2006, my husband Jorge and I welcomed our twin boys, Andres and Emilio, into the world. I can see today how many blessings we have truly received.

My first good news was when I got past my first trimester and a blood test revealed an extremely low likelihood of Down syndrome. (I'm 35, so we were a little concerned about this.) My second breakthrough was when I got past the 32-week period. (Babies born earlier than this often can have great difficulties). My third breakthrough was when a final ultrasound revealed my boys had reached full term size, quite a feat for a twin pregnancy. My fourth breakthrough was delivering both of my sons with minimal interventions. My greatest gift of all was that both of my sons were born healthy. They took to breastfeeding easily, and we were able to take them home within 48 hours after delivery.

The bond that has been cemented between my children and I is unbreakable. It really helps that they are so cute! Everything I do today keeps them in mind: from driving more carefully, to the type of music I play, to the company I keep and the commitments I make.

Every day is a new beginning for our family: we'll see a new smile or new awareness in their faces, or even hear a new kind of cry. I'm continually amazed with the incredible turn my life has taken. So, if you want to have a baby, keep an open mind because anything is possible. I'm in awe that after only 3 months with my babies, the adventure has just begun.

Bibliography

Hundreds of books and articles were reviewed during the writing of this book. Because of space constraints, the editors have chosen to list a representative sampling here.

Abernathy, Sarah, "Herb-Nutrient-Drug Interactions: Facts You Need To Know." Healthy Healing. 2003

Balch, James, M.D. and Mark Strengler, N.D. Prescription for Natural Cures. 2004

"Bed Sharing with Siblings, Soft Bedding, Increase SIDS Risk," National Institutes of Health, May 2003

Bevinetto, Gina, "5 Ways to Recreate the Womb," americanbaby.com, 2006

Bone, Kerry, FNIMH, FNHAA, "Tribulus for Men & Women: Part 2," Nutrition & Healing, Sept. 1999

Boyles, Salynn, "Anxiety during pregnancy increases ADHD Risk," WebMD July 16, 2004

Busser, Maggie, "Exploring Waterbirth," Balanced Living Magazine LLC, 2002

Chappell LC, Seed PT, Briley AL, Kelly FJ, Lee R, Hunt BJ, Parmar K, Bewley SJ, Shennan AH, Steer PJ. Effect of antioxidants on the occurrence of pre-eclampsia in women at increased risk: a randomised trial. Lancet. 1999;354:810-16

Chopra, Deepak, M.D. and David Simon, M.D. A Holistic Guide to Pregnancy and Childbirth. Three Rivers Press, 2005

Dallinga JW, Moonen EJ, Dumoulin JC, Evers JL, Geraedts JP, Kleinjans JC. Decreased human semen quality and organochlorine compounds in the blood. Human Reprod 2002; 17:1973-1979

DeNoon, Daniel, "Rate of Preterm Birth Hits New High in U.S.," WebMD, Sept. 9, 2005

Dodt, Colleen K., Natural Babycare. Storey Pub. 1997

Donaldson-Evans, Catherine, "Acupuncture: A Cure for Infertility?" FOX News, April 26, 2005

Dwek, Laurie Budger, "Poor Prenatal and Infant Nutrition Connected to Health Problems," Natural Foods Merchandiser, August 2003

"Electromagnetic radiation and miscarriage," the John R. Lee, M.D. Medical Letter, March 2003

"False Labor, False Vs. True Labor," American Pregnancy Association, © 2000-04.

Felder, Lyn and Shiva Rea, "Yoga for Moms to Be," Yogajournal.com, 2006

"Folic acid, Zinc Supplements May Help Men with Fertility Problems," WebMD, March 20, 2002

Harper, Barbara, "Waterbirth Basics: From Newborn Breathing to Hospital Protocols," Midwifery Today, Issue 54, Summer 2000

"Heart gone haywire blamed in some infant deaths," American Heart Association, 11/19/2002

"Higher SIDS Risk Found in Infants Placed in Unaccustomed Sleeping Position," National Institutes of Health News Feb. 2003

Hitti, Miranda, "Paxil's Birth Defect Warning Strengthened" WebMD, Sept. 27, 2005

Ishikawa H, Ohashi M, Hayakawa K et al. Effects of Guizhi-Fuling Wan on male infertility with varicocele. Am J Clin Med 1996; 24:327-31

Karp, Harvey, "Curing Colic: The 4th Trimester, the Calming Reflex & the 5 S's," 2001-2006 Pregnancy.org, LLC

Karp, Harvey, Happiest Baby on the Block: The New Way to Calm Crying and Help Your Baby Sleep Longer. Bantam Books, 2002.

Kemper, Kathi, M.D., M.P.H. The Holistic Pediatrician Second Edition. Quill 2002

"Labor & Delivery: What You Need To Know About Cesarean Birth," March of Dimes, Dec. 2005

Li, DK, et al, "A population-based prospective cohort study of personal exposure to magnetic fields during pregnancy and the risk of miscarriage," Epidemiology 2002; 13:9-20.

Maccorkle, Jill, "Homebirth Under Fire," Mothering Magazine, March/April 2003

"Massage Delivers Babies," Natural Health, November/December 1998

"Medical Tests in Pregnancy," Birth International, 1997-2005

Meletis, Chris, N.D. & Liz Brown. Enhancing Fertility. Basic Health Publications, 2004

"Men, Your Fertility Clock is Ticking," WebMD, Feb 5, 2003

Mindell, Jodi, Ph.D. "Sleep Concerns: Ear Infections," BabyCenter, Dec. 2003

"Mother's DHA Levels Predict Maturity of Baby's Brain," The Natural Foods Merchandiser, Nov. 2002

"No Benefits from Episiotomy, Study Finds," consumeraffairs.com, May 3, 2005

O'Mara, Peggy, Mothering Magazine's Having A Baby, Naturally: The Mothering Magazine Guide to Pregnancy & Childbirth. Atria 2003

Page, Linda, Ph.D., Traditional Naturopath. Healthy Healing 12th Edition: A Guide to Self-Healing For Everyone. Healthy Healing Pub. 2004

"Postpartum depression," Mayoclinic.com

"Pregnant with twins: What are the risks?" BabyCenter LLC. 1997-2006

"Prenatal nutrition" Whole Foods Magazine, July 1998

"Reasons You Might Need to Abstain from Sex During Pregnancy," BabyCenter Editorial Staff 1997-2005.

"Recognizing and Responding to Colic," dummies.com 2006

Romm, Aviva, C.P.M., A.H.G. The Natural Pregnancy Book. Celestial Arts. 2003

Rubin, Rita, "Battle lines drawn over C-section," USA Today, 2005

Rusch, Elizabeth, "New Baby Basics," Plum Magazine First Edition, 2005

Schwartz, Richard MD, "All About Rh Disease," Discover Communications, 2005

Sears, William. The Fussy Baby: How to Bring Out the Best in Your High-Need Child. Little Brown & Co., 1996.

Sherman, Neilia, "Do Multiples Equal Cesarean? A Guide to Vaginal Twin Births." iParenting.com 1996-2004

"Soaring Cesarean Section Rates Cause for Alarm," American College of Nurse-Midwives, Jan 13, 2003

"STD Surveillance 2002: STDs in Women and Infants," Oct. 2004

Tierra, Michael, L.Ac., OMD, A.H.G. and Leslie Tierra, L.Ac., A.H.G. Chinese Traditional Herbal Medicine, Vol. 1 & 2, Lotus Press 1998

"Toxic Landfills May Cause Birth Defects," WebMD, Jan 24, 2002

"Treating Diaper Rash," drgreene.com, April 20, 1996

"Useful Herbs in Pregnancy," Earth Mama Angel Baby 2002, 2003

"Uterine Fibroids," BabyCenter Medical Advisory Board, 1997-2005

"Warning: Teflon Can Cause Birth Defects & Infertility," Environmental Working Group, March 28, 2003

Weed, Susun. The Wise Woman Herbal Childbearing Year. Ash Tree pub. 1986

White, Linda, M.D. "Wise Use of Herbs and Vitamins During Pregnancy," ChildbirthSolutions 2000-2005

Woolven, Linda "Herbal Allies for Pregnancy," Mothering Magazine, 2006

References

Infertility Resources

The National Infertility Association - National Helpline: 888-623-0744, http://www.resolve.org

InfertilityCentral.com connects couples with information, support and solutions.

The American Society for Reproductive Medicine (ASRM) is an internationally recognized leader in the field of reproductive medicine, http://www.asrm.org/

Pediatric Illness & Conditions

The March of Dimes is a not-for-profit organization whose mission is to improve the health of babies by preventing birth defects, premature birth, and infant mortality, http://www.marchofdimes.com

America's Baby Cancer Foundation (ABCF) raises awareness of baby cancer, and helps fund research. Telephone & Fax (562) 433-4512, http://www.babycancer.com

Children's Health and Parenting Links

Mothering Magazine, http://www.mothering.com/

iVillage's Pregnancy & Parenting Info, http://parenting.ivillage.com

http://www.babycenter.com

Twins & Multiples

National Organization of Mothers of Twins Clubs, Inc, http://www.nomotc.org

Adoption: An option for beginning and growing families

Adoption.com is committed to helping as many children as possible find loving, permanent homes, http://www.adoption.com

http://www.adoptuskids.org - A project of The Children's Bureau, part of the Federal Department of Health and Human Services. 888-200-4005.

Foster Parenting

National Foster Parent Association - The only national organization which strives to support foster parents, and remains a consistently strong voice on behalf of all children. (800) 557-5238, http://www.nfpainc.org

Child Abuse Prevention

Prevent Child Abuse America - builds awareness and provides education to everyone involved in the effort to prevent child abuse and neglect. 800-CHILDREN, http://www.preventchildabuse.org

Loss & Bereavement Support

The Hygeia Foundation, Inc. & Institute for Perinatal Loss & Bereavement - http://hygeia.org

Herbal Education & Resources

Clayton College of Natural Health - http://www.ccnh.edu

East West School of Herbology - http://www.planetherbs.com

Product Resources

All One, 719 East Haley St., Santa Barbara, CA 93103, 800-235-5727

Aloe Life Intl. P.O. Box 710759, Santee, CA 92072

American Health, 2100 Smithtown Ave., Ronkonkoma NY, 11779, 800-445-7137

Barleans Organic Oils, 4936 Lake Terrell Rd., Ferndale, WA 98248, 800-445-3529

Baywood Intl., 14950 N. 83rd Pl., Ste.1, Scottsdale, AZ 85260, 800-481-7169

Crystal Star Herbs, 121-B Calle Del Oaks, Del Rey Oaks, CA 93940, 800-736-6015

Diamond/Herpanacine, 145 Willow Grove Ave. #1, Glenside, PA 19038, 888-467-4200

Earth Mama Angel Baby, 9866 SE Empire Court, Clackamas, OR 97015, 503-607-0607

Fairhaven Health, 1200 Harris Avenue, Suite 403, Bellingham, WA, 98225, 360-671-0859

Fresh Baby, 616 Petoskey Street, Suite 202, Petoskey, MI 49770, 866-403-7374

Flora, Inc., 805 East Badger Road, P.O. Box 73, Lynden, WA 98264, 800-446-2110

Green Foods Corp., 320 North Graves Ave., Oxnard, CA 93030 800-777-4430

Health from the Sun/Arkopharma, P.O. Box 179, Newport, NH 03773, 800-447-2229

Herbal Answers, Inc., P.O. Box 1110, Saratoga Springs, NY 12866, 888-256-3367

Herbs for Kids, 1441 West Smith Road, Ferndale, WA 98248, 800-232-4005

Home Health, 2100 Smithtown Ave., Ronkonkoma NY, 11779, 800-445-7137

Imperial Elixir, P.O. Box 970, Simi Valley, CA 93062, 800-284-2598

Jagulana Herbal Products, Inc., P.O. Box 45, Badger, CA 93603, 888-465-3686

Jason Natural/Earth's Best, 4600 Sleepytime Dr., Boulder, CO 80301, 800-434-4246

Lane Labs, 25 Commerce Drive, Allendale, NJ 07401, 800-526-3005

MagiaBella, 5742 W. Harold Gatty Drive Salt Lake City, Utah 84116, 800-448-2095

Maitake Products, 1 Madison St. Bldg. F, East Rutherford, NJ 07073, 1-800-747-7418

Merix Health Care, 18 E. Dundee Rd. #3-204, Barrington, IL 60010, 847-277-1111

Moon Maid Botanicals, 535 Tall Poplar Road, Cosby, TN 865-217-9713, 877-253-7853

Mother's Intuition, 866-450-4MOM (4666), www.tummyhoney.com

Motherlove Herbal Co., P.O. Box 101, Laporte, CO 80535, 970-493-2892

Mychelle Dermaceuticals, Box 1, Frisco, CO 80443, 800-447-2076

Natracare, 14901 E. Hampden Avenue, Suite 190, Aurora, CO, 80014, 303-617-3476

Nelson Bach, 100 Research Dr., Wilmington, MA 01887, 800-319-9151

New Chapter, 90 Technology Dr., Brattleboro, VT 05301, 800-543-7279

Noveya, 19 Be'er Sheva, Jerusalem, Israel, 94507, 201-675-9170

Nutrabella, PO Box 1722, Palo Alto, CA 94302-1722, 800-95-BELLY

NutriCology, 2300 North Loop Road, Alameda, CA 94507

Prince of Peace, 3536 Arden Road, Hayward, CA 94545, 800-732-2328

Pure Essence Laboratories, Inc., P.O. Box 95397, Las Vegas, NV 89193, 888-254-8000

Pure Planet, 1542 Seabright Ave., Long Beach, CA 90813, 562-951-1124

TenderCare Intl., Inc., 3925 North Hastings Way, Eau Claire, WI 54703, 800-344-6379

UAS Labs, 9953 Valley View Rd., Minneapolis MN 55344, 800-422-3371

Wakunaga of America / Kyolic, 23501 Madero, Mission Viejo, CA 92691, 800-421-2998

Well in Hand, 5164 Waterlick Rd., Forest, VA 24551, 888-550-7774

Wellements, 3925 E. Watkins St., Suite 200, Phoenix, AZ, 85034, 800-255-2690

Xlear, Inc., P.O. Box 970911, Orem, UT 84097, 877-599-5327

Yoanna Skin Care, P.O. Box 610072, Redwood City, CA 94061, 800-366-4617

Index